Going to Hell in a Handbasket

A Collection of Reader-Submitted Medical Stories

Kerry Hamm

Disclaimer:

Names, locations, and portions of the details included in this book have been altered to protect the privacy of those involved.

<u>Warning:</u>

This edition features light profanity that may be offensive to some readers. The profanity has been used sparingly and in each instance the usage was included in the submission. I have chosen to leave some of these words in to emphasize portions of the stories.

By now, I am sure you are all too familiar with my *Real Stories from a Small-Town ER* series, which were collections of stories told to you from my time as a registration clerk in Ohio. If you are new here, don't fret! You don't have to worry about a 'certain order' for *any* of my books, including this one!

I have since moved on from the hospital scene, but that hasn't stopped readers from submitting stories of their own experiences from the medical field. Over time, I have received hundreds of stories-some funny, some sad, some downright scary or grotesque-and have worked with my readers to bring these stories to you in a follow up to my last *Real Stories* volume.

If I've learned anything from writing my series and compiling this book, it's that none of us are alone. We're all proof that we've seen some seriously messed up things out there, right? We have seen the good. We've seen the bad. We've seen the downright vile and disgusting. And then, we've seen the humor in these situations and we've been fortunate enough to share them with one another. There is a certain peace in knowing that as no matter how crazy we feel, we have formed solidarity amongst ourselves, knowing that for every bad day you've had, others have had them too. We have worked through the challenges of getting up and facing another drug seeker, another child abuse case, another young death, and another 'how the heck did that even happen?' moment together. You guys are not alone, and this book reaffirms that.

Several of the stories have been edited to bring you clear-cut and clean versions of tales submitted by loyal readers. I have done my very best to edit out hospital and town names, and in some cases my submitters wished to withhold their initials and other details from publication or requested that I edit stories for grammar/spelling. Some stories have been edited for length. I do my very best to preserve a reader's humor and emotions, as well as capture the reader's personality when I edit these submissions.

Though some of the stories in this collection are horrifying, I am glad none of us are alone in what we've witnessed or experienced.

<u>Cheat Sheet</u>

Some readers have been confused about terms used in this series. Here's a quick list to help you out!

LEO: Law Enforcement Officer

ETOH: shorthand for Ethyl Alcohol or Ethanol; commonly used to describe intoxicated individuals

Bus/Rig/Truck: Ambulance

M.D.: Medical Doctor

R.N.: Registered Nurse

MVA: Motor Vehicle Accident

EMS: Emergency Medical Services

EMT: Emergency Medical Technician

PD/FD: Police Department/Fire Department

D.A.: District Attorney

BOLO: Be on (the) Lookout

DCFS/CPS: Department of Children and Family Services/Child Protective Services

SNF: Skilled Nursing Facility. This can be a nursing home or one of many facilities for patients in need of supervised care

AMA: Against Medical Advice

LWBS/LBT: Left Without Being Seen/Left Before Triage

LOL: Little Old Lady

Half Baked

We received a half-assed report from EMS at 03:30 one weekday, telling us to expect "too much to tell you, but trauma to the scalp and substance abuse."

Right off the bat, I was absolutely positive we were going to get someone who'd shot up a bunch of heroin and then got his brains beat out with a ball bat. It wouldn't be the first time we'd received a patient like that. In fact, that seems to happen at least once a month around here on the night shift.

When I saw on the cameras that EMS pulled in the bay, I went to a trauma room and waited for my patient. It felt like transport was taking longer than usual, but I wasn't in the mood to go find out what was keeping them.

As I was waiting, I heard banshee screams from down the hall.

"Oh, hell no," I said to myself, as I started grinding my teeth. This was the last kind of patient I wanted to deal with, especially since we'd all been so busy that night that none of us had gotten even half a second to eat or use the bathroom.

EMS rolled my patient in the room. She was restrained, but that didn't stop her from trying to kick and scratch at the medics.

"Better get you some help in here," one of the medics said. "I'd make sure not to let her out till she comes down."

"From what?" I asked with a groan, as the patient started hissing and making racket like alley cats fighting.

"Roommate says she took some E (ecstasy) and smoked some pot. I guess she had already been drinking. Roommate says she's had at least three shots of tequila and two mixed drinks."

"And nobody thought to stop her from doing all that?" I asked.

The medic shrugged. "Roommate was messed up, too."

"Shocking," I replied sarcastically.

The patient was shrieking so loudly that I could hardly hear the medics as they tried giving me the patient's vitals.

Now, the weirdest part wasn't that the patient was drugged out of her mind. It wasn't that she was loud or combative.

No. The weirdest part of this admission was seeing that part of the patient's scalp was hanging by centimeters of bloody flesh that looked like it'd fall off at any second. Matted in a section of the patient's long, beautiful hair was a metal beater that attaches to a hand mixer. (Yes, a hand mixer that you use in the kitchen.) Much to my surprise, it didn't appear to be actively bleeding, but the patient was partially scalped.

We got the patient transferred to an ER bed. She bit a medic in the process, and when our doc heard the commotion, he demanded that security be notified and then ordered her to be masked.

As we tried to mask her, however, she looked at me, screamed bloody murder and called me a 'devil centaur,' right before she blew chunks down the front of my pants and all over my favorite shoes. She then gasped and attempted to break free from her four-point restraints, began wheezing, and coughed so hard that she puked again. The doctor saw all this and said that because she was at risk for aspirating, we couldn't mask her.

In a way, I'm glad we didn't mask her because her temperature was reading between 104 and 106, and we landed on those numbers as we could barely get the thermometer swiped across her forehead. When I placed my hand on her arm, it felt like I was holding my hand to the front of my oven after it's been turned off a while. Security and extra staff arrived, held her down, and we were able to get a temp of 106.7.

For a few minutes, we tried for an IV, but the patient was going berserk. She was totally convinced we were all 'devil creatures' and that we wanted to harvest her organs, at least from what I could understand from her wild rants. We swapped out our female nurses for three burly orderlies holding her legs, security holding her abdomen, and our male RNs holding her upper quadrant. We had to work at lightning speed to get an IV started, and then we strategically placed cold compresses around her body to lower her temperature.

"Hey," someone called to me.

"What?"

"She has a visitor in the lobby."

"No. Not a chance in hell anyone's coming back here with her like this," I snapped.

"Registration said it might be her mom. I don't know."

I sighed and figured I should go out front and talk to the mom. There wasn't much I could really do at the moment, and the patient was being watched, so I could consider it a break.

When I went to the lobby, 18,000 people rushed to me because they thought I was there to call visitors back or to call the next patient. I had to put my hands up like I was a crossing guard, and then I had to yell that I was looking for Ms. Doe's mother.

At first, nobody came forward.

"Did you just call back there and tell someone my patient's mom is out here?" I asked a frazzled registration clerk.

The girl at the counter pointed down the hall to two women who were pacing in front of the water fountain. As I neared the women, I realized they weren't too much older than the patient, who was about 15 years younger than I was. These women just *looked* older, clearly due to drugs, alcohol, and excessive tanning.

I try not to be too judgmental of how patients or visitors dress in the ER—after all, you're not coming to the hospital to participate in a beauty pageant. These women, however, had itty bitty shredded crop-top tank tops covering their stubby breasts. One was wearing mesh booty shorts and the other had on a mini skirt so short that I could *literally* see her vagina as she struggled to remain upright in front of me. It was clear both women were under the influence. Ms. Booty Shorts seemed more coherent and functional than Ms. Mini Skirt, so I directed my questions to her.

15

"Do you know how much Ecstasy she took?" I asked.

"I dunno."

The woman in the short skirt moved her in closer until her nose was touching my cheek and whispered, "I've never met an angel before."

"Why don't you go sit down?" I asked. It came out as more of a snide order, but I didn't care. I was annoyed.

Ms. Booty Shorts laughed and said, "I don't know what all she took. I know we smoked some wet, though. And then we did the other shit."

I sighed.

"Well," I asked, "what happened to her head?"

Ms. Mini Skirt started twirling around in circles and when she stopped, she was so dizzy that she fell into the wall, slid down the wall, and when her ass hit the tile floor, she pissed herself. A river of urine flowed across the hall.

A few witnesses started commenting loudly in disgust.

"Oh, come on!" I yelled. "It's not enough that your friend is in there, doped out of her mind and hurt, but you're pissing yourself in public and showing your snatch to the whole free world?"

I kid you not, the woman in the skirt looked up at me with a thick sliver of drool hanging from her bottom lip to her stomach, and then she said in a slur, "You're, like, not very cool."

She then passed out and I yelled down to registration to get someone up front to help me.

"We brought her cookies," Ms. Booty Shorts said to me, referring to my patient. She looked around for a minute and then giggled, "Oh. They must be at the apartment."

I cursed under my breath and then asked, "Is that how she got the beater stuck in her hair?"

Ms. Booty Shorts cackled and nodded. "She wanted to, like, bake cookies. But then, like, her hair got caught and there was, like, a lot of blood. So, like, I took her downstairs and called, like, that number."

"Idiot," I muttered to myself as I knelt and checked for a pulse on Ms. Mini Skirt.

I helped my coworkers get snatch-flasher back to a room, and then I went to check on my patient who was screaming, "This place is on fire! Help! There's a fire!" at the top of her lungs.

The rest of the story isn't that eventful. We called in a surg-consult for the patient's scalp. Our surgeon on site consulted another surgeon at a place about an hour out. Both surgeons agreed that the best course of treatment was to attempt to reattach as much of the patient's scalp as possible, but it turned out that there was a portion that our surgeon deemed too damaged to reattach. He did his best.

Officers arrived shortly after we moved Ms. Mini Skirt to the back because Ms. Booty Shorts started stripping in the waiting room. She and Ms. Mini Skirt were found in possession of illegal substances and were placed under arrest. Ms. Mini Skirt was handcuffed to an ICU bed and stayed for observation. My patient, I think, was admitted for a few days.

I have no clue what happened to my patient after she was discharged. I can only hope she realized that drugs were ruining her life and sought treatment. I also hope her friends came to the same realization. Unfortunately, I can't tell you whether these women kicked their habits.

-M.O.-L.

Location withheld at request

<u>Wrap It Before You Tap It</u>

When you work in the ESD (Emergency Services Department), you sometimes think you've seen it all. Then you have idiots like the two patients I'm about to tell you about come in, and *then* you've seen everything.

Our day shifts are busier than our evening and overnights combined. We easily clear 200 patients per day on my shift, and that's just on an average day. To say we don't have a lot of time for petty B.S. is an understatement. Our administration listened to staff feedback and added 10 fast track rooms. These rooms help a great deal, but they don't solve our problems. We are among the busiest ESDs in the country, and it's exhausting.

One afternoon, we received what the registration department was calling a '2 for 1.' Once I had the two in one of our triage bays, I learned we could not place these patients as such. Had they come in for something like a cold, yeah, we probably could have treated them in the same room, no problem.

The female patient informed me she was experiencing vaginal tenderness, pain, and bleeding. She said these complaints were consistent with trauma. In fact, those were her exact words. I opened a can of worms by casually asking if she worked in the healthcare field, to which she replied that she did.

"I'm a vet tech," she said. "Thanks for acknowledging that I'm actually part of this industry."

I wanted to roll my eyes, but that little voice in my head told me to play nice. After all, she probably had a role in saving lives, just not human lives.

"Tell me about this trauma," I said.

Her male companion still hadn't said a word. His face was red, and he was sweating, but the woman was the one doing all the talking, so whatever. You snooze, you lose.

"Well," she said, looking around as if she had a camera crew following her every move, "it's kind of private."

"The more you can tell me, the better," I said. "I won't judge, and everything you tell me is private, except for informing your doctor."

She said, "We were fooling around. That's how it happened."

"Regular intercourse?" I asked. I was tired and hungry. I was on autopilot and my tone reflected this.

"Um…" she hesitated. She thought for a second. "Well, the sex was normal, if that's what you mean. But the other part…"

I kind of raised my brows but didn't say anything.

"Well, we didn't have a condom," she said, "but we still wanted to do it."

Again, I didn't say anything. I honestly didn't care at this point. I just wanted her to tell me what happened and get on with it, so I could get the two to rooms, check off with their assigned nurses (if needed), and speak with a doctor (if needed).

"So, we used a Ziploc bag," the woman said to me.

I blinked hard, shook my head, and asked, "You what? You used a Ziploc bag as a condom?"

The woman nodded and explained, "But we didn't go for very long because it hurt real bad."

"Uh…" I said.

"And now he can't get it off," she said.

Wait, what?

"He can't get the bag off? What?" I asked.

The woman nudged her partner and said, "Go on, show her."

Before I could object, the male stood, dropped his jeans, and exposed what I can only describe as a swollen purple and blue chubby snake. Most of the bag had been cut or torn away, except for scraps of plastic…That were held against the patient's penis with a zip-tie that was cutting off his

23

circulation to the point that portions of his penis were blackening.

"Oh my God, what did you do?" I yelled, jumping up from my seat.

A security guard posting in the hall moved to just outside my bay and asked, "Is everything okay in there?"

"Uh, yeah," I stammered.

"Why did you do that?" I asked the male patient.

He shrugged and said, "We didn't have a condom."

"So, you go buy one or something!" I exclaimed. "You don't use a zip-tie. Oh my."

The female threw a fit when I informed her she could not be placed in the same treatment room as her partner. She calmed some after I explained she could join him after she was examined and treated, if her partner agreed to have her in his room. He assured me this would be okay, and the couple gave each other a very long, very awkward kiss that involved heavy usage of tongues.

From what I understood, the female patient was advised to take it easy for a week or so, just to allow her superficial vaginal lacerations to heal.

The male, on the other hand, was in our ESD for quite some time because it, apparently, proved difficult for multiple nurses and doctors to remove the zip-tie from the patient's appendage. It was so tight that it was digging into his penis and staff couldn't wedge the scissors in between his penis and the thick plastic band to cut the device from the patient. Our ESD doctors called someone from surgery for a consult. Luckily, the surgeon had an idea. She kept a tiny pair of folding scissors on her person because she knits in her free time, including on her breaks. Thankfully, because these scissors are much smaller than what the ESD shears can access quickly, as opposed to calling Central Supply and waiting 45 minutes to receive the wrong order.

It did take the surgeon another 15 minutes to cut through the zip-tie, and she nicked the patient's appendage twice. His wounds were practically non-existent, and according to office chatter, the patient probably wouldn't have minded even a nasty cut or two, as long as someone could remove the tie from his penis.

Honestly, I suppose I have to give this couple kudos for attempting to practice safe sex, but in the future, I do hope they purchase condoms. I know it's probably terribly wrong of me to think, but I also hope these two never reproduce.

-I.G.

Texas

"Ouch!" I said to my female patient presenting with a nasty burn to her eyelid and eyebrow region. "How'd you do that?"

Her response was the very last thing I expected to hear, well, ever.

She said sheepishly, "I was trying to curl my eyelashes with my curling iron."

-N.S.

Alabama

Doggone

I am not a nurse, nor do I work in the healthcare field. My sister (14-year ICU veteran, 5-year ER veteran), however, got me hooked on your books. She's been pressuring me to send you this story, but I was pretty sure my husband would kill me for doing so. My sister and I finally agreed that what he doesn't know won't hurt him.

Okay, so let me take you back to the hottest day of summer, when everything that could go wrong did go wrong. First, I overslept. Then, on my way to work, I was side-swiped by a girl who'd been distracted by her cell phone. Even though I called my new boss (who was the biggest jerk I'd ever met) and explained that I had been in an accident, he fired me. He said I didn't give a timely notice that I would be late because I didn't call him at least an hour before my shift started, like the rules in our employee handbook stated. I guess working there for 11 years meant nothing to that man, who'd seemed hellbent on getting rid of all the old employees and hiring fresh. (Yes, I hired an attorney. Unfortunately, we are considered an at-will state as far as employment goes, so basically anyone can get fired for anything, unless discrimination or something like that is proven.) When officers arrived on scene to take a report of the wreck, I was given a ticket because I realized I'd forgotten my purse at home. That meant I didn't have my driver's license, and my insurance information was also in my purse because I had just switched insurance companies the day before. The other driver was cited, but her problem became my problem because she was uninsured.

My husband was supposed to be getting off work soon, so I called him and told him what happened. He said to go to the gas station across the street from where my wreck had happened, and he would be there soon. He wasn't there soon. The idiot clocked out from work, drove home, and fell asleep. I didn't have my purse with me, so I couldn't pay anyone to drive me home. I tried calling a bunch of people, but nobody would answer. I'm not kidding; I called my husband 14 (FOURTEEN!) times before he finally picked up the phone.

"Did you forget something?" I asked him.

"I don't think so," he said.

"You freaking forgot to pick me up!" I yelled. "I've been at this gas station for two-and-a-half-hours!"

You know what he said?

He said, "Oh."

No, "Hey babe, I'm sorry." No, "Oops." No, "My bad."

Just, "Oh."

I waited another 25 minutes for him to come pick me up, and then we went back home.

To top it all off, our central air decided to break from the time my husband left the house to the time we got home. My husband doesn't know anything about fixing that kind of stuff and neither do I, so I called a technician, who told me the company was backed up with work orders and the soonest anyone could come out to the house was the next day. Our house becomes a sauna without central air, so my husband and I were both dripping in sweat within an hour of coming home. We were so uncomfortable that my husband couldn't sleep.

When he suggested we go to Lowe's and buy at least one window air conditioning unit, I practically jumped for joy. We went to Lowe's, bought two window units, and drove home.

Not one to ever make a fuss about having to do anything, I grabbed one of the units from the bed of the truck.

"I'll get that," my husband said. "You just go inside and watch TV or something."

I argued with him about how I wasn't a delicate flower and all that crap, and I started carrying this heavy box up the driveway.

Well, about halfway to the house, I lost my grip on the box and dropped a 41-pound air conditioner on my foot.

I was wearing flip flops.

I cried.

A lot.

My husband drove me to the emergency room, where we were for about four hours before I was discharged with a cast on my broken foot and had to learn how to use crutches.

Of course, since we hadn't installed the air conditioners, it was about 130-degrees in our house when we got home. Our poor chihuahua was lying on the bathroom floor, right in front of the fan. She shot me daggers when I had to move her out of the way to pee.

Now, I think it was just habit at the time, because this definitely wasn't in the front of my mind, but I used an ovulation strip while I was in the bathroom and excitedly yelled to my husband, "It's time!"

I didn't necessarily want to have sex, but we'd been trying for a year to get pregnant, and since I wasn't getting any younger, we weren't wasting any time. So, broken foot or not, we were going to make it work.

I heard one of the new air conditioners kick on from upstairs, and then I heard my husband running across the house like a madman.

By the time I got out of the bathroom and into the hallway, my husband was completely naked at the top of the stairs. He was standing there, waving his ding-a-ling like a helicopter propeller, because men seem to think that's the way to turn a woman on.

"You know I can't come up there," I said.

"But there's no air conditioning in the guest room," he whined.

"Well, get down here and install it, and then let's go," I said.

I added, "Hurry. The medicine they gave me is making me tired."

"I'm coming!" he said in a giddy tone. I swear, this man's been having sex since he was 16, and 25 years later he's still as excited as a teenager when he knows he's gettin' some.

Well, my husband was acting like a fool, getting loud and still swinging his penis around, which made our dog think that he wanted to play. I know what you're probably thinking here, so I'll tell you that no, my dog did not bite my husband on the penis or testicles.

Instead, as the dog was running up the stairs, my husband was running down the stairs. Since the dog was on one step lower than my husband was, my husband decided to yell, "Geronimo!" and attempted to jump over the dog, to the step under the dog.

That didn't go to plan.

My husband tumbled down the stairs, knocked me over (I was screaming and crying because he landed on my cast), and was doubled over on the floor, also screaming and crying.

"Did you break your foot?" I asked.

I don't exactly know why I asked that. I guess, with the way things were going, I just assumed that would be our luck, to both end up in the emergency room with a broken foot within hours of each other.

When he didn't answer, I asked, "Gary, what'd you hurt?"

"My balls," he choked through heaving sobbing.

"I'll call Sandy," I said, as I hobbled towards the living room, where my cell phone was.

"Do NOT call your sister!" my husband yelled.

"She's a nurse," I said. "She can look at you and see if you need to go to the hospital."

"I don't want your sister looking at my balls," he screamed.

"Stop being a baby," I said. "It's not like she's never seen a naked man before."

"Just call 911."

"And pay for an ambulance?" I asked. "You want to pay for an ambulance, when we could just have Sandy drive?"

My husband reached down and then started screaming a shrill scream that you hear young girls do in horror movies.

"What's wrong with you?" I yelled. "Stop screaming like that. I just broke my foot, and I didn't scream like that!"

"One of them's gone!" he shrieked. "One of them's GONE, Leslie!"

"One of what?" I asked, before realizing to what he was referring.

Then I gasped and asked, "Are you sure?"

"I think I'd know if one of my balls was gone!"

"Well," I asked, "where'd it go?"

My dumb ass started looking around the tile floor while my husband, holding himself up by the knees and one palm on the floor. His other hand was cupped over his testicles. Well, testicle.

"I can't feel it," he cried. "Oh my God. Oh my God. I lost my ball."

"You're gonna be okay," I told him.

"Call 911!" he wailed. "Hurry! Call 911!"

The 911 call went something like this:

"911, what's your emergency?"

"My husband fell and said one of his testicles disappeared."

"His testicles?"

"Yeah. I don't know what happened, really, but he fell and said he can't feel one of his testicles anymore."

"Is he bleeding? Did he hit his head?"

"No, just his testicles."

(My husband was screaming from the background, "Tell them to hurry, Les! I'm really scared!")

"Is your husband bleeding from his groin?"

"Are you bleeding from your groin, Gary?"

"I don't know! What's taking so long? Oh my God, I need help!"

"I heard him, ma'am. Give me your address, and I'll send a unit to your residence."

My husband refused to let me help him get dressed, so I gave up on trying to help him and must have fallen asleep on the couch. So, EMS arrived to a naked man crying on the hallway floor, a chihuahua barking, and a woman with a broken foot fast asleep. My husband and I were both sweaty, too, so I have no idea what those paramedics were thinking.

We all loaded in the back of the ambulance (the paramedics helped me get in), and we went to the hospital, where my sister was assigned as my husband's nurse. I guess calling her wouldn't have helped, anyway. She explained her relationship to my husband and another nurse was assigned to my husband.

Well, the first nurse felt around my husband's testicular region and said she couldn't feel the testicle floating around, so the doctor came in and ordered a urine test to test for blood. That came back clean, so they came in with a machine that reminded me of an ultrasound machine, and they said my husband's testicle had ascended into his inguinal canal.

Man, you would think my husband was being burned alive by how much he was screaming while we were in that ER. My sister actually had to come in at one point and tell my husband that if he didn't calm down, they were going to have to give him meds to force him to calm down. I mean, he was freaking out about *everything*. He started worrying about not being able to have kids, was worried about what the guys at work would think...You name it, he was freaking out about it.

Well, the emergency room doctor said he couldn't do anything else except schedule my husband for surgery, so they transferred my husband to the Clinical Decision Unit. They said they use that unit as overflow for the ER, for people needing blood transfusions and scheduled stuff like that, or for people like my husband, who really didn't need to go to ICU or anything, but they weren't ready to be discharged from the hospital.

I slept in the waiting room while my husband was in surgery. I don't think it took very long at all, but when I went in his recovery room, he was coming off the anesthesia and he must have been hallucinating because he kept talking about *The Brady Bunch* like he was actually a member of the family. He was asking all the nurses about the Brady family and wanted to know if they (the Brady's) were in the waiting room. When I tried to explain to him that they were not at the hospital, he started crying. A doctor came in to check on him and started laughing so hard that he had to leave the room.

Since I didn't have a car at the hospital and couldn't drive home even if I wanted to, I waited with my husband and then my sister took me home. She helped me install the air conditioner in the guest bedroom and I think I slept for a good 11 hours.

My husband was discharged the next afternoon, and he swore me to secrecy on the whole thing. He didn't want anyone ever knowing what really happened. In fact, when he called off from work, he told them that he had a yardwork accident. The doctor wrote him a note to be off work for the remainder of the week, just to 'recover from a traumatic experience.'

Just to fill you in, we didn't end up having much sex that cycle or while I had my cast on, but we eventually got around to it and I ended up having twins (when my OB-GYN showed us the ultrasound monitor, my husband fainted and had to get three stitches on his chin), and I ended up being a stay at home mom, while doing some light telemarketer work from home.

-L.K.

Indiana

<u>I Will Follow You</u>

K.S. shares the most ridiculous 911 call she's answered. It goes something like this:

K.S.: 911, please state your emergency.

Caller: Hi, yes, I overslept.

K.S.: Are you experiencing a medical emergency?

Caller: I don't think so, but I will be if I can't get to my interview on time.

K.S.: Ma'am, are you aware that you dialed 911?

Caller: Yes.

K.S.: Ma'am, are you in danger right now?

Caller: Huh? Uh, not that I'm aware.

K.S.: So, you called to report that you overslept?

Caller: Yeah. I'm supposed to be at this interview in 10 minutes, but I know for a fact that I've never been able to get to that side of town without taking at least 15 minutes.

K.S.: If this is not a medical emergency—.

Caller: Well, I'm not sick or anything, but I need you to send someone to my house.

K.S.: Why?

Caller: Because if you call them to my house, I'll just follow them to my interview.

K.S.: Ma'am?

Caller: Well, I know you guys do escorts because I've seen videos of cops giving people escorts to the hospital and stuff. And I've seen them leading funeral processions.

K.S.: Ma'am, none of our emergency services offer escorts to interviews.

Caller: But I saw it on TV. I know you do. I saw these cops escorting an ambulance one time.

K.S.: Officers typically only do that when there's been an emergency.

Caller: The word 'emergency' is subjective, don't you think?

K.S.: Ma'am, are you aware you can be ticketed and even arrested for using 911 for non-emergencies?

Caller: But I need to get to this interview.

K.S.: Then I suggest you call a taxi, ma'am.

Caller: But I don't want to pay for that. It's going to cost a lot to get across town. Plus, I know they take the longest way possible to try to scam people out of money.

K.S.: Ma'am, I'm ending this call. Please consider this a warning not to call 911 unless you're experiencing an emergency.

One minute, eight seconds later...

K.S.: 911, please state your emergency.

Caller: Uh, yes. I'm having, uh, extreme pain in my, uh, right lower abdominal quadrant.

K.S.: Ma'am, if you are not experiencing a true medical emergency, you will be wasting valuable resources that we could use on patients experiencing legitimate emergencies.

Caller: I'm not lying, though. I need the police or someone to come to my house.

I told the patient I could arrange that, and then I dispatched the nearest EMS crew, along with the nearest LEO team.

According to EMS, the caller became irate when EMS refused to act as an escort for her. She was arrested for assaulting a medic, so I think it's safe to say she did *not* get the job for which she planned to interview that morning.

The strangest thing I've ever seen inserted into someone's body is a pair of cement hands clasped in the prayer position.

The hands were a little smaller than real hands, and we couldn't get them out in ES, so our 'extreme worshipper' had to go to surgery.

-K.W., M.D.
New Mexico

Giddy Up

I work the overnight shift and during one slow shift, I decided to take a paid break to step outside for a cigarette and to check my text messages. I lit up and started going through messages from my family, when I heard a loud clopping noise coming from down the road. I heard a few cars honk, too, but I was more concerned with that clopping sound. I just couldn't figure out where it was coming from, exactly, and I wasn't quite sure what it was.

Thinking maybe it was one of the 18-wheelers that drive that busy road daily, I went back to my phone and hopped on Facebook.

I heard a horse whinny, and I looked up. From what I could make out, a female rider wearing a set of silk pajamas was directing this huge black horse off the main road and onto hospital property. She was riding that horse through the parking lot just like she was driving a car through the lot.

Of course, my first reaction was to get on Snapchat and send a picture to all my friends. The caption was, 'Look at this lady riding a horse through the parking lot at 03:00, LOL.'

I guess it never really crossed my mind to inform security or the police about this. I mean, yeah, it's pretty unusual to see someone riding a horse through the city unless they're in a parade or something, but I didn't think there was a law against it or anything. Also, she wasn't hurting me, so hey, ride on, lady.

I finished smoking and went inside. I hadn't been paying attention to the horse or its rider. The intake clerk was off doing who-knows-what, and I didn't have a desire to talk to anyone in back, so I didn't tell anyone what I'd seen.

Well, there I was, sitting at the registration center, trying not to fall asleep, when the woman rode her horse up to the ED entrance, hopped off and tied the horse's reins to a no-parking sign, and then I saw the woman zig-zagging toward the entrance.

The closer the woman got to the door, it became painfully obvious that she was impaired. She couldn't walk in a straight line and almost fell a few times. Her pajama pants were muddy and wet from the knees down. When she arrived at the registration center, I could see the buttons on her pajama blouse were misaligned. The woman's eyes were bloodshot, what I instantly knew to be Fireball whisky radiated from her body, and she slurred as she spoke.

"I need to see a doctor," she told me.

"Were you in an accident?"

"I ain't had no accident," she replied angrily. "Why are you accusing me of stuff? You don't even know me, and you're accusing me of doing something wrong?"

She inserted expletives in between nearly every word she said.

"Ma'am," I stated calmly, "your appearance suggests you were in an accident."

I motioned to her elbow and said, "You're actually bleeding. Are you here to be seen for an accident?"

She dramatically drew her right arm to her chest as if she planned to give a prim and proper speech at an eloquent dinner party. She slurred, "If you must know, I fell off my horse and landed in the trough, thank you very much."

"And is that why you're here?" I asked, as I picked up the phone to call the back and hopefully track down the intake clerk.

"Why are you so nosy?" the woman snapped. "Do you ever cook my breakfast?"

I chuckled and asked, "What?"

I didn't plan on laughing at what she had said, but it happened. And boy oh boy, did it piss her off.

This lady started screaming at the top of her lungs that I was discriminating against her because of her ethnicity, which made zero sense because she and I were of the same ethnicity.

Someone in back answered the phone, and after I asked the person if he could send the intake clerk to the front, I hung up the phone and dialed the switchboard operator to request security.

The belligerent woman at the registration center took her anger to the next step when she heard me ask the operator to page security.

"Now you're calling the cops on me?" she shouted. "I ain't ever done anything to you, but you're gonna call the cops on me?"

"Ma'am," I said in a tired, dry tone, "I need you to lower your voice and stop cussing at me."

"This is America," she snapped. "You might want to read up on this little thing called Miranda Rights."

"You mean the thing that says you have the right to remain silent?" I asked.

"You can't tell me to stay silent!" she shrieked. "I am a woman, and I have been oppressed for too long, and I will not be silent!"

The intake clerk walked in during another profanity-riddled rant and the poor girl, who was a shy girl who'd just graduated from high school and had the unfortunate luck of being hired for the position with the highest turnover rate in the ED area, shot me a wild look that begged, 'Please don't make me do this.'

"I can register you to be seen now," the clerk said to the belligerent woman, offering her a polite smile.

"I didn't have to register last time I was here," the woman snapped. "What is your problem? You think that just 'cause you get to wear colorful clothes that you can tell me what to do? 'Cause it don't work that way, you smug little bitch. That's right, I called you little. What're you gonna do about it? Nothing. That's right, I said nothing."

Knowing full well the clerk wouldn't speak up for herself, I said, "Ma'am, everyone has to register to be seen in the emergency department. And please stop cussing at us. We are just trying to help you."

"If you wanted to help me," she shouted with a cynical tone, "you would get me Taco Tierra. You don't really care about me. All you people are the same. You get paid to pretend to care."

Security arrived right around the time the woman began destroying the lobby. The guard asked me to call law enforcement, right before he attempted to prevent the woman from picking up and throwing another chair.

The guard lost his train of thought in the middle of this, and he asked, shocked, "Is that a horse out front?"

The newly hired intake clerk was shaking when she asked me, "Does this happen a lot?"

"Uh," I said, "not really."

The officer managed to convince the drunk woman to sign in, and he personally escorted her to an empty exam room. We all thought this was the best course of action because law enforcement needed to confront this woman about her behavior and ensure she could get home (or wherever) safely.

Since I lucked out and didn't have to triage the patient, I sat up front with the intake clerk and waited for officers to arrive.

"Did you know there's a horse in the parking lot?" one of the officers asked me.

I nodded and said, "Your woman back there rode it here."

"She rode a horse to the hospital?" the officer asked with a laugh.

"She sure did," I said. "Better buckle up, guys. That woman is about to take you for a ride."

My gut feeling was correct. Within about 30 seconds of the officers disappearing to the back and (undoubtedly) entering her room, I could hear her screaming and demanding narcotics.

The next thing I knew, the ED doors that separated the exam area from the lobby area flew open and the woman stormed out. Her top was open, exposing her bare breasts and a flat belly with a belly ring.

This woman flipped the intake clerk and me off and shouted, "Screw you! Screw this hospital! I'm never coming back here! You messed with the wrong woman. My dad is the Prime Minister! I'm gonna tell him what you did, and he's gonna fire you!"

The woman removed her pajama blouse and threw it to the floor. She then exited the ED and was trying to climb on her horse as officers emerged from the treatment area.

"Where'd she go?" an officer asked me.

I nodded toward the entrance.

"Damn it," the officer groaned. "I knew tonight was gonna be like this."

"Why's that?" I asked.

He said, "Because it's my first night back from vacation."

All three officers went outside and since one of them stood in front of the ED doors, the sensor detected a presence and wouldn't close. I could hear almost everything.

"Ma'am," said one of the officers, "I need you to come down from the horse."

"I have rights," she argued. "You can't tell me what to do. I ain't done nothing wrong."

"Ma'am," the officer repeated, "please come down from the horse."

"Why?" she demanded. "I'm not doing anything wrong!"

The officer was growing tired of her backtalk and said, "We have reason to believe that you're under the influence. You are breaking the law right now. Now, please get off the horse."

"No," she said.

This argument went on for about 30 seconds before the officer reached up and grabbed the woman's arm.

As he tried to pull her off, she fought with all her might and said in a strained shout, "Just let me ride this horse, damn it!"

She kicked her horse in the sides and the horse started to move, but its reins were still tied to the sign.

"If you don't come down by the time I count to three," the officer said, "I'll have no choice but to tase you."

As you can probably guess, one, two, and three came and went without the woman obeying police orders, so the taser was deployed and instead of falling off the horse and landing on the ground, she rolled off the horse's back and was hanging with her foot stuck in part of the horse's gear. Officers assisted the woman off the horse and placed her on the ground, where she was flopping around and screaming so much that I honestly couldn't tell she had even been tased.

We had to get a few people up front to help get her inside. She went through a med clearance and officers ran a drug and ETOH screen. Unsurprisingly, the woman tested positive for alcohol and methamphetamines.

Her bad luck didn't end there.

Because she was intoxicated and attempted to flee on horseback after abusing staff and going on a demanding rant, the woman was arrested for a DUI and animal cruelty. The police department called in someone who owned a trailer, and they loaded up the horse. I guess they took it to another woman's farm, since they couldn't exactly take it to the vehicle impound.

Oh, and guess what? It wasn't even her horse! An officer told me that a few hours after they arrested the woman, a guy she used to work for called in a report of a stolen or lost horse, so they returned the horse to its rightful owner.

-Name and location withheld at request

Fright Night

I was taking my first break of the night, and it was much needed. We'd seen codes, ODs, and pediatric abuse patients back to back for five hours, and the whole time, I had to poop. It's hard enough to do my job without my body pressuring me to have a bowel movement, but it's much harder when I have to actively remind myself, 'Wait it out.'

I walked around the hospital to find a bathroom that would be 1.) Vacant, 2.) Out of the way, so nobody else would come in, and 3.) That had the updated fixtures, as opposed to some of the facility bathrooms that still had sinks from 1943 and those paper towel dispensers that always jammed when you pushed the lever down. I finally found the perfect bathroom and entered a stall.

This is where it gets sort of weird. See, ever since I've been a child, I just *can't* have a bowel movement unless I take my shoes off. I've come a long way, because my mom laughs and tells stories of when I was a toddler, and how I stripped down to my birthday suit when I had to use the bathroom. Don't worry, I didn't get naked in the bathroom stall. I slipped off my clogs and set them neatly by the stall door.

I had just began going, when I felt a tickle on the top of my right buttocks. I have long hair that sheds quite a bit, so I figured a strand must have come loose and was the source of the tickling. I kind of wiggled on the seat to knock the hair loose.

Seconds later, I felt the tickle again. And this time, I could tell it was moving. I knew it wasn't a hair.

Because I was still using the restroom, I kind of leaned forward and grabbed at the tickling spot. I felt something moving in my hand, and when I opened my hand to exam, I fuzzy spider crawled from my palm and ran up my arm.

In mid-poop, I hopped up from the toilet, screamed a bunch of obscenities, and then felt a stab through the arch of my foot, which made me scream even louder. As I was wildly flapping my arms, trying to get the spider off of me, I noticed two things:

Firstly, my foot was bleeding through my sock enough to leave splotches on the floor. Secondly, there were now at least 50 tiny fuzzy spiders running all over the toilet seat, and I realized I had them all over my scrubs. Some were even in my underwear. I screamed again and tried to pull up my scrubs, while I was using a free hand to open the lock on the stall door.

In addition to stepping on what I determined to be a key to my locker, I tripped over my shoes, fell forward out of the stall, and hit my chin on the sink. I hit it so hard that the sink cracked. I guess I bit my tongue in the process, so I had bloody saliva running out of my mouth as I sobbed, and my chin was also bleeding.

The worst part is I didn't even have my pants pulled up all the way, and I still had to poop.

No, no. Strike that.

The *worst* part is that a security guard heard me screaming and crying. I never heard him knock, so when he entered the bathroom, my pants and panties were only pulled up to cover half of my butt. He saw the stupid Patrick (from Spongebob) tattoo that I had gotten when I was a teenager. That's a totally different story and alcohol was involved.

He kind of looked around and told me that he thought someone was getting beat up in the bathroom, but I had to tell him what had really happened. He then called switchboard and told the operator to notify the emergency room of an injured employee, and I had to be treated for a puncture wound to my foot, as well as have my chin gash glued.

I guess all the spiders came from an egg sac that had hatched. When HR was investigating my work comp complaint, they became curious of how an egg sac could have remained under the toilet seat for that long, and it was determined that none of the janitors cleaned that bathroom for over a month because they said nobody ever used it. Well, I used it, but I'll never use it again.

I got sent home that night, and then I took a few days of PTO because I was too embarrassed to go back.

All my coworkers still tease me about that incident. They call me things like 'Spider Woman' and 'Arachnophobia.'

--K.C.

Kentucky

<u>Citizen's Arrest</u>

Years and years ago, I took my kids to the park. My oldest was about four at the time, and my youngest had to have been about six-weeks-old.

The place was pretty busy. The playground area wasn't too far from the walking trail, so not only were there kids playing all over the place in front of me (and all the other mothers, grandmothers, and sitters), but there was also a lot of traffic to my left, where all the joggers, dog-walkers, and speed-walkers were.

I was breastfeeding my daughter and watching my son, but I was zoning out, too, so I'm not sure how long the commotion had been going on...but I heard screaming and looked over to the walking trail to see a man closed-fist hitting a woman.

I was appalled, of course. I was shocked and disgusted and angry and all of those emotions. But I was also an exhausted night nurse with one baby on my boob and another baby who was (thankfully) so wrapped up in playing with his little friends that he wasn't paying attention to the assault in progress.

This was back when cell phones first came out. When I say cell phones, I mean think back to when they came in a huge black zipped bag. I only knew one person who owned one, and that person wasn't at the park with me. I kind of looked around to see if there was a male who could step in, but the only males I saw were the assailant and an elderly man who was sitting with his wife on a bench across the way. As I scanned my surroundings for anyone who could help, I noticed almost everyone shared the same expressions of disapproval and fear over what this man was doing to this woman.

While one woman was telling everyone that she was going to find a pay phone to call the police, the elderly man struggled to stand up. He relied heavily on his cane, a thick piece of wood that was carved with designs and shellacked, giving it a shiny appearance. He was already out of breath when he was halfway to the assault, so I stood up and called to him as I moved closer. I didn't want him trying to get involved and end up getting injured.

I guess the elderly gentleman didn't hear me or chose to ignore me, because he approached the man who was beating the woman.

"Excuse me?" the elderly man said to the woman-beater.

The assailant turned his head for one second, laughed as he gave the elderly gentleman a once-over glance, and then said, "Mind your business, old man."

He then punched the woman so hard that she fell down. Her face was swollen and already bruising. Her lips were so swollen that they looked like pictures you'd see of plastic surgery gone wrong. There was blood everywhere.

"Young man?" the elderly gentleman said again. "Young man?"

"Didn't I tell you to mind your own business?" the abuser screamed, as he turned to face the elderly man again.

As soon as he whipped around to face the elderly gentleman, the elderly man hit the assailant in the testicles with his cane. The abuser dropped to his knees. Unfortunately, the elderly gentleman lost his balance and also fell. He hit his head and was bleeding.

I honestly didn't have a choice at this point, so I handed my infant to a woman who'd been sitting next to me, and I hurried to the elderly gentleman's side. I applied pressure to his gushing head wound and yelled for someone to find help after he told me he was taking blood thinners.

As if there wasn't enough drama happening in the park already, the abusive man got up and pushed me away from the elderly gentleman. I was covered in blood, could hear my newborn crying, and my son was running towards me, screaming, "Mommy! Mommy!"

The abusive man then kicked the elderly man in the ribs, and the elderly man began crying. His wife was trying to make her way to us, but she wasn't very mobile, either.

Thankfully, a jogger passed us and was carrying mace. She sprayed the assailant in the eyes and another (male) jogger who was running with a big dog pushed the assailant over to the side, away from people, and made him sit on the ground with his hands behind his head until police officers arrived. We all learned that the abusive man was married to the woman he was beating. She told officers that she wanted to tell her husband that she wanted a divorce and thought that telling him in a public place would stop him from hitting her like he hit her at home.

Two ambulances arrived and transported the elderly gentleman and the assault victim to the hospital. Medics asked me if I needed transport, but aside from all the blood (that I had to wash off by using one of those spigots you see at campsites), I was okay physically. Mentally and emotionally, I was extremely shaken up. I had to sign a bunch of papers and give my account to officers before I could leave.

I didn't think that I'd see any of the parties involved in that incident again, but a few months later I saw the abuse victim. She was a patient on one of my shifts, but my coworker was assigned to her. I guess the woman called off the divorce because her husband swore he wouldn't hit her again, but she was being seen that night because her husband beat her so badly that she had to go to surgery.

-K.W.
Illinois

<u>That Sucks</u>

"Hey," shouted our unit clerk around two in the afternoon, "can someone take this call? I can't understand what this guy's saying, but he's freaking out."

I was voluntold to answer.

"RN Smith," I said. "Can I help you?"

I have to say, I really wasn't expecting a teenage boy to reply.

His breathing was heavy and erratic. He sounded as if he was possibly crying. It was hard to hear him at times because there was a loud whirring noise in the background.

"I-I-I saw this thing that said you could use a v-vacuum to j-j-jerk off," he said in sheer panic, "b-but I can't... Oh my God, I think I need an ambulance or something because it won't come off. If I call 911, they're gonna call my mom at work. I need help! I-I can't get it off! I s-swear. If you help me get it off, I'll never do it again. I swear."

71

It took me a second to process everything that I was hearing.

"You have a vacuum stuck on your penis?" I asked.

Boy, say that out loud if you ever need to get everyone's attention, let me tell you what.

"I-I can't get it off. I don't know what to do. It hurts. P-p-please, you gotta help me."

At this point, the poor kid was sobbing and choking on his words so much that I could hardly understand him.

"You need to calm down," I said. "You're going to give yourself a panic attack or something."

"But it's stuck. It h-hurts. Oh my God, my dick's gonna get ripped off and my mom is gonna find out. She's gonna kill me."

"Honey," I asked, "have you tried turning the vacuum off?"

"Oh my God," the kid said hysterically, right before I heard the whirring noise come to an abrupt stop.

"Did that help?" I asked.

"Oh, thank you God. Thank you so much. Oh my God, thank you. Thank you so much."

"How 'bout you don't ever do that again," I suggested.

The kid sniffled and coughed and then finally said, "I-I won't," before hanging up.

Now, some of my coworkers have questioned the authenticity of the complaint, but I'm telling you that I work with scared and injured patients day in and day out. I'm almost positive that was a real emergency for that kid.

I've never had anything like that before, and I'm actually kind of glad my supervisor made me answer that call.

-F.N.
Michigan

__Babysitting__

I was the nearest unit to respond to a call in a residential area. According to dispatch, a concerned neighbor witnessed a group of young children playing with an infant outside. She requested a welfare check.

To be quite honest, I was thinking that the call was probably someone getting her panties in a bunch. I mean, honestly, these days we want kids to get out of the house and play, but when they do, we have a lot of Busy Betties calling 911 over the kids being too loud at the park or using chalk on sidewalks. Our department even receives calls regarding unaccompanied and/or unsupervised minors. Then, we'll get there and find a few pre-teens riding their bikes to the park or something—performing innocent, legal activities—and there's nothing to write home about. You just can't please people these days, I tell you.

I drove to the caller's address. This is something else I should tell you. See, most of the time, when anyone calls 911 or any type of first responder service, we don't have the address of the actual scene of crime, fire, or medical emergency. We often have no choice but to ride up to the initial caller's home and speak to that resident, or if we're lucky, dispatch will be able to get descriptions of the emergency's location from the caller (the house with the red shutters and blue door, for example).

In this situation, I had no visual of young children playing with an infant. The caller was on her porch, however, and she flailed her arms to get my attention.

"Ma'am," I asked, "did you just place a call to 911?"

This woman was in her 80s and was no taller than my 10-year-old daughter.

"Those kids," she said, pointing across the street, "have a baby. Now, I don't know where they got that baby. I suppose where all babies come from, but someone's gotta be missing that baby."

"Did you see where the kids took off to?" I asked.

She nodded excitedly and said, "Well, yes. They ran around back. Now, I was going to go over there and take the baby from them, but you see, I can't make it down the front steps."

She motioned to her porch steps, and then to her knees. "They just give out, anymore. I can't even check my mail. My daughter has to come over if I need to go anyplace. Like Dr. Smith's office, where I need to go this Thursday. You see, he said I need a bi-annual. I told him that Dr. Doe never pressured me to have a bi-annual. He only saw me once a year. Before that, he said only come in when I felt ill. Sad that he passed. He's survived by his wife. Now Jane, she makes the best turkey pot pies in the county. She's won five blue ribbons."

Have you ever been around someone like that? I swear, half of my calls are spent standing around, trying to find the polite time to interrupt someone.

I heard children making loud noises, so I excused myself. The caller stood on her porch and watched as I crossed the street and walked between two vacant homes. One of the homes was condemned, and that in itself had me concerned. From the sounds of the children's playful screams, they sounded young. Surely, what the caller had witnessed was a child playing with a baby doll.

When I walked around back, I saw five young children chasing each other through a half-dead yard, up porch steps and around the porch, and all over the place. These kids were no older than six-years-old.

What was more troubling is that I could hear an infant, and there was just no way the cries could belong to a toy's recording.

"Hey, guys," I said, announcing myself.

All but four of the children froze in place. The fifth child, a boy, took off running. I called after him, but he was gone, and I was more concerned with the children present.

"Do your parents know you're out here playing?" I asked.

None of the children answered me.

I moved slowly between the group, searching for the crying infant. After a few seconds, I stopped at the far side of the rickety porch and looked down. Under the porch, behind some cracked and discolored lattice, there was an infant lying in a pile of soggy leaves and dirt. Spiders and soil bugs scurried over her face and fleece onesie that smelled of urine and feces.

"That's my sister," one boy said to me. "You can hold her if you want to."

I immediately picked the baby up, tried to wipe the dirt from her skin, and pulled the onesie from her, leaving her in a sagging soiled diaper. It was far too hot for her to be outside, especially in that type of outfit. Her crown appeared to be sunburnt, as well as her face and hands. I figured this baby couldn't have been more than three-months-old.

"She wants a bottle," said a girl from the group. "But John forgot the bottle."

"It was an accident," the boy said. He started crying and asked me if I was going to take him to jail.

"No," I told him. "I am definitely not taking you to jail."

"Are you taking me to jail?" another little girl asked.

As I held the infant, I sat on the porch steps and explained to the children, "Policemen don't take kids to jail. We're here to help you, not take you to jail."

I said, "Do your mommies and daddies know you're playing outside right now? Do they know where you are?"

"Well, we were supposed to go to the park," said one of the girls.

The other boy in the group said, "Stop! If you tell, we'll get in trouble."

"Nobody's gonna get in trouble," I said. "Not from me. But you see, this house isn't safe to play at. It's really old and falling apart. We don't want anything bad to happen to anyone, right?"

The boy in the back said, "Jason Smith was at the park."

"Who's Jason Smith?" I asked.

"He's in second grade, and he's really mean," one of the girls replied.

"So, you all left the park because Jason Smith was being mean?"

Three of the kids nodded.

"And what about your mommies and daddies? Were they at the park, too?"

"I don't have a mommy or daddy," one of the girls told me. "My grandma takes care of me."

"Oh," I said. "Was your grandma at the park, too?"

"No," she said. She explained one of the boys and the other girl from the group were siblings. They were given permission to go to the park that was one block from their apartment complex. On the way, they stopped at this child's house and asked if she could go to the park. They met the boy with the baby and my runner at the park.

"Well," I said, "I think we need to get some of you home. I bet you're real hungry, huh?"

I called in for backup and social services and waited for both to arrive. Social services brought chips and juice barrels for the kids. I relinquished custody of the infant to social services after giving my initial statement and moved to talk to the infant's brother.

"Your sister is really hungry," I said. "Can you tell me where you live, and we can go get a bottle?"

He shook his head.

"She can't eat the chips like you can," I said. "And she's real hungry. Don't you want her belly to be full, too?"

He nodded.

"Why don't you tell me where you live," I said, "and we can go get her a bottle to drink. We can get her a new diaper and pick out a pretty little dress and—."

"We can't go," the boy interrupted me. He reached in his pocket and showed me a silver watch. He pointed to the face of the watch and said, "We can't go back until the big hand is on the one-two, and the little hand is on the three."

"Why's that?" I asked.

He looked away.

"You can tell me," I said.

He wouldn't answer any of my questions related to home until I bribed him with two quarters. He then informed me that 'Johnny,' his mother's 'special friend,' was at home, and he couldn't go home until three, because that's when Johnny left. According to the child, his mother 'fell asleep' a lot, and then Johnny would 'do bad things' to the boy and his sister, so the boy began leaving soon after waking. He told me that on that morning, Johnny threw a plate at him, so he forgot to grab the bag that had 'all the baby stuff' in it.

Thankfully, the child agreed to go with me to his residence. I promised him that he didn't have to go inside, that he could stay with one of the nice ladies from social services who followed us in another car and had the infant in custody.

The home was a single-family home and appeared to need TLC. I knocked three times before a man with a haggard appearance and alcohol on his breath opened the door.

"What do you fucking want?" he snapped at me.

"Sir, I'm looking for the parent or guardian of a young boy and an infant."

"What for?" he asked.

"I'd like to ask her a few questions."

He snorted and said, "She's busy."

"At any time today," I asked, "were you the responsible party for the children?"

"They ain't my kids," he yelled. "I ain't taking care of shit."

"Is the mother here?" I asked.

"Told you," he said, "she's busy."

The man then pulled out a crack pipe from the pocket of his tattered shorts, and he attempted to smoke while I was standing approximately two feet in front of him. I entered the home at this point and saw a woman in her late-twenties passed out on the foyer floor.

Johnny was placed under arrest for a slew of drug-related charges, and EMS responded to an overdose for the kids' mother.

As the investigation continued, it came out that Johnny was the mother's boyfriend/drug supplier. Nobody seemed to know who the kids' biological father was. The kids' mother routinely used drugs in the presence of her children and there were closed files from social services that showed the boy's teachers and even some neighbors had complained that the children seemed neglected. Both kids tested positive for trace amounts of various drugs. Johnny was also charged with several molestation-related charges, after it came to light that the 'bad things' he did involved inappropriately touching both the young boy and the infant.

Luckily, social services tracked down the families for the other children, and we even found out who the runner was. No charges were filed against those parents and/or guardians, but social services opened case files and conducted routine visits to ensure the children were safe.

I have to say, I am incredibly thankful someone called 911 to report this incident because the infant was admitted to our local ER for dehydration and a few other minor complaints. Overall, she was in good health, but she needed a bit of attention after being out in the heat since seven that morning.

I don't like to talk about this much, and I couldn't bring myself to explain my day to my wife. She still doesn't know the details of this day. She knows something happened and kind of caught what it was about because some of it made it to the local newspaper, but I can't open up to talk about it. Writing to you is the closest I've been to seeking therapy for this situation, and I want to thank you for listening and keeping my information private.

-Name and location withheld at request

Now You See Me

Local PD brought in this kid for underage consumption one night. They found him wandering around a neighborhood, and when they tried to stop him, he ran and fell. We treated him for a skinned knee. Officers basically gave him a warning and asked us to hold him until they could track down his parents.

This kid was around the age of 16 and had never touched alcohol before (according to him). From what we could tell, he was invited to a party and was told to leave because the cool kids thought he was a loser. On his way out, he stole a bottle that was filled half-way with Jim Beam, drank it in the park, and was so hammered that a breathalyzer probably would have been off the charts if the kid had even so much breathed in its direction.

I hate to say it, but I guess I could understand why the cool kids thought our patient was a loser. He cried when we cleaned up and bandaged his knee. As he would talk incessantly about Pokémon and some video game called Gorogoa, he must have used his shirt to clean his glasses about a thousand times. He just seemed a bit dorky, but he was polite and funny.

I was in his room, cleaning up from when we'd treated his knee, when the patient told me he was pretty heavy into magic and wanted to be a magician after he graduated. He told me that his big plan was to skip college, hitchhike to Vegas, and try to get a job at a casino as a headliner. I just laughed and nodded.

At first, I thought the kid was pretty good. I mean, yes, his tricks were simple and overdone. They were the cliché tricks that we'd expect all magicians to pull off during amateur hour or at a grade-school talent show. He pulled a coin from behind his ear, and then he bit the coin in half, waved his free hand in front of it, making it whole again. He then reached in his pocked and started pulling out one of those endless ropes made out of mesh-like hankies.

He was talking my ear off, so when he asked, "Hey, wanna see me disappear?" I just kept my mouth shut and shrugged.

He stood up from the bed and yanked the sheet off. He held the blanket with his fingertips and moved it in front of him, until I could only see his fingertips.

"Ready?" he asked.

"Sure," I said.

The patient then dropped the blanket and tried to use the falling sheet as a distraction. I guess what was *supposed* to happen is that I was supposed to be watching the sheet fall to the floor while the patient bolted from the bed to the door. I guess I was never supposed to be the wiser.

But, that's not what happened.

The patient tried to run to the door, but instead of running through the doorway, he ran into the glass *next* to the door and broke his nose. He immediately started shrieking.

Of course, the kid's parents walked up to the room just in time to see their kid crouched on the floor, catching all of this blood in the palm of his hands.

I put my hand on the patient's shoulder and started to ask if he was okay, but I think he was embarrassed because he screamed at me, "Get away!"

The patient's mom walked in and asked accusingly, "What on earth did you do to my son?"

I tried to explain what happened, but she wasn't hearing it. She demanded that she speak to our House Supe, so we paged him, and our doctor inspected and treated the patient while I sat with Charge and told my side of the story.

Thankfully, the kid was placed in a mental health treatment room, so there were cameras in each corner. When the Supe came down, we (Charge, the Supe, the patient's parents, the doctor, and I) were all watching the video that showed the events up to the patient breaking his nose.

"Again with that stupid magic stuff?" grumbled the patient's father.

"Well," mom snapped, "it's your dad's fault for buying him that kit for his birthday."

"I didn't see your parents buying him a football helmet."

"John," the wife sighed, "you know very well that my parents would have, had they not died."

While the parents were bickering, my colleagues and I kind of shot each other looks of bewilderment.

And there it was, the moment of truth. Charge advised me not to speak, so we watched in silence as the patient lifted the sheet in front of his body.

Our Supe opened his can of Coke and started chugging.

On screen, the patient took off across the room, and then-BAM!

Coke shot out of the Supe's mouth, landed all over our Charge, and soda was foaming out of his nose. He was choking and laughing so much that we couldn't understand him when he tried to apologize to the parents. In fact, he had to put his hands up to excuse himself until he could gather composure.

The patient's mom was pissed and said that all the video showed was that I was in the room and failed to properly restrain her son to keep him from harming himself.

"Jane," her husband said, "he knocked himself out last week with a book tied to the ceiling fan. The boy's destined to have his ass kicked a few times. You should just be thankful that he's doing it to himself and he's not getting it from the kids at school."

Mom and dad took the patient home and housekeeping went in to clean the room. Thankfully, the rest of the night was uneventful, but it was fun while it lasted.

-R.M.

Arkansas

Can You Smell What the Neighbor's Cooking?

I once responded to a call regarding a property boundary dispute. On scene, I was rather unhappy to learn that the homeowner called 911 because he could smell his neighbor's barbeque from inside his house.

I maintained professionalism and suggested to the homeowner that he close his window if he did not wish to smell his neighbor's barbeque.

The homeowner said he appreciated that I took the call to come out, we said our goodbyes, and I walked back to my patrol car.

As I was pulling out of the drive, I saw the homeowner climb over his chain link fence with a fire extinguisher under one arm and a mop (the kind with the strings) in one of his hands.

I cussed a little and then told dispatch he may want to send an additional unit, just in case the situation evolved out my control.

I didn't exactly walk, but I can't say that I ran, either. I think I'd take a few steps by walking, and then I'd jog for a few steps. Once I heard a female screaming, I picked up the pace.

When I arrived in the neighbor's backyard, the male who'd called 911 was using the fire extinguish on his neighbor's grill. A female was standing near the neighbor's back porch, yelling for the subject to stop.

The homeowner attempted to stop the honorary fireman by taking a swing at him, but the subject dodged, dropped the fire extinguisher, picked up the mop, and started swinging (string-side toward his victim).

Do you know how insane and stupid I felt screaming, "Sir, put the mop down!"?

I mean, I am a parent, and anyone with kids can tell you parents yell some stupid stuff. "Stop licking the dog. If you put one more M & M in the toilet you're going to bed early. Stop telling your brother to smell your farts."

I have literally said all of those things, and yet ordering the subject to drop the mop at three in the afternoon in a nice subdivision has got to be in the top 10 of dumbest things I've ever said in my life.

"I do not like bratwursts!" my subject screamed in response. "I hate the way they smell! My entire house smells now!"

"We're not even cooking brats," yelled the female.

"Sir! Put the mop on the ground now!"

The subject took a few more swings at his male neighbor. He did hit him once before the victim grabbed hold of the mop and a struggle ensued. This resulted in the subject bumping into the grill and knocking it over. Red and gray charcoal briquettes scattered on the ground, along with two ribeye steaks and a few hot dogs. My victim then fell and braced himself for the fall with his hands. He screamed as his palms hit those hot briquettes and he jumped up.

Just as he jumped up, his neighbor swung the mop and hit the subject in the face. It was a combination of shock and force that knocked my subject back to the pile of briquettes.

This time, the subject was slow to move.

I ordered the neighbor to drop the mop. He complied without protest.

Honestly, I didn't feel that the neighbor was in the wrong. All I saw was a man defending his property and wellbeing following a crazed attack.

The subject, on the other hand, was placed under arrest while we waited for EMS. I followed the ambulance to the hospital, where the subject was treated for minor burns to his hands and arms.

You'd think that he would've have gotten the fight knocked out of him, but he didn't. After nurses bandaged his hands, he apparently thought the bandages resembled boxing gloves and he took a few swings at me.

This subject was not under the influence of alcohol or drugs. He was just an asshole.

-B.F.

Ohio

In a Pickle

We operate in a rural area and respond to calls within a county that has a population of roughly 15,000 people in several small towns spread out over hundreds of miles. Like most crews, we do respond to non-emergent calls placed to 911, and we still have our frequents. However, those calls are a small, small percentage of our routine responses. Typically, I would say that in one month, 98% of our calls are truly emergent. We normally deal with trauma cases, as we see an outstanding number of vehicular accidents and/or farming accidents. We also see a great number of falls and the like.

On the night in question, we were dispatched to a drive-in movie theater approximately 40 minutes from our station. A town closer to the call has a station there, but they receive such low volumes of calls at night that they only work during the day and part of Friday and Saturday nights. It was after the time they packed up, so my partner and I were complaining the whole drive. We were also flying down this country highway, doing probably about 90-95.

"Only good thing about this," I said, "is that we can bullshit our time and watch part of a movie."

"And hot dogs," said my partner. "They have the best hot dogs."

We didn't quite catch what dispatch was saying because something was going on with our radios, but we expected to see a bloodbath because there are a lot of accidents where the drive-in theater lane meets the highway. Semis and other vehicles fly down that road, and even in daylight it's hard to see if there's anyone coming as you pull out of the theater parking lot area. I still don't know why nobody's thought to put a warning sign or something out that way, but whatever.

Anyway, we got out to the movie theater area, and there was no wreck to be found. We turned off lights and sirens, drove down the lane that opened to a huge open field where all the vehicles were parked, and we parked our rig next to the concession stand.

"I'm gonna go call the station and see what the hell we're supposed to be responding to," I said to my partner.

He nodded and said, "I'm gonna go get a hot dog while you're doing that."

We both got out and started walking up to the concession stand counter, when we heard a female screaming at the top of her lungs, "Over here! Hey, ambulance guys! Over here!"

She must have had a good set of lungs on her because we could hear her over the 50-something speakers in the field. You know, they were garbling words and I'm sure most people were picking up the movie's audio with their car radios, but the speakers were still pretty loud.

"I want my damn hot dog," my partner grumbled. "Making us drive all the way out here. This better be something good, or I swear to God…"

Most people continued watching the movie as my partner and I walked between rows of cars. Some people yelled at us to move out of the way. So sorry that someone's medical emergency is causing you to miss eight seconds of a movie you paid $5 to see, right?

When we finally met up with the woman who'd been screaming, we realized she was a young girl, probably fresh out of high school. Her car was a hooptie, with a back seat filled with empty water bottles and fast food bags and wrappers. Another young female was squirming in the passenger seat, sobbing and breathing heavily.

"What happened?" I asked.

"Would you guys shut up?" a man to the side of us yelled. He was lying on a blanket on top of the hood of his truck. "I'm trying to hear the movie."

"John," my partner yelled back, "if you can't hear the movie with two speakers next to you, that ain't our problem."

"She had an accident," said the driver of our parked vehicle. "We tried to get it out of there, but we can't. It was supposed to be a joke."

I kind of blinked and waved my head and open palm-up hands around like John Travolta in *Pulp Fiction*. "What was? You haven't told us what the problem is yet."

It was a quiet part of the movie, and I mean almost dead silence. You could hear some people talking from their cars or around their cars, and you could hear the generators from the concession stand running. There was an eerie hum in the air from a barely-audible stream of static coming from all the speakers and the radios operating in unison.

The girl in the passenger seat broke that silence by screaming, "I have a pickle stuck in my vagina!"

We could see people turning around from their car seats and people on the lawn were looking around, trying to see who screamed that.

"Come again?" my partner asked.

"It's her fault!" the patient yelled, pointing angrily at the girl who was standing there, talking to us.

"Well, it's not like I forced you to do it," the girl snapped back.

"Let's save the arguing for later," I suggested. I leaned in the car through the driver's side and asked, "How did you get a pickle stuck inside of you?"

"I don't know!" the patient yelled. "It turned sideways or something. I can't get it out."

"No," I said, laughing a little. "How did you... Why did you stick a pickle in your vagina in the first place?"

"Because she dared me to see if it'd fit," the patient replied.

"Look, bitch," said the driver of the car, "I didn't hold you down and make you put it up your vag. I said I wondered if it would fit up *someone's* vagina. And I didn't even say yours. And, you know what? I said that as a joke. I couldn't believe you were stupid enough to do it."

The girls started arguing with each other.

"Get out of my car," the driver screamed.

"I can't get out," the patient yelled back. "I need this thing out of me."

The driver ran around to the passenger side of her car, yanked the door open (after a minute or so of trying because the handle was broken), and she snatched the patient by the hair and dragged her out of the car. Our medical run then became a mission of breaking these two up as they started beating the crap out of each other. People around us were screaming for the girls to shut up and move out of the way.

"I'm so glad I get paid nine-dollars an hour to deal with this kind of crap," my partner grumbled, as we struggled to separate the young ladies.

The patient pulled out of my grip, turned, and shoved me in the chest. She demanded, "Take this thing out of me now!"

I shook my head and said, "We don't do anything like that. If it's stuck, we're going to have to get you in the ambulance and transport you to the emergency room."

"Will they be able to get it out?" she whined.

I shrugged. "Probably. I mean, I would imagine they'd be able to get it out fairly easy, but that's just my opinion."

"Then let's go," the girl ordered.

I hate when people act that way. Like, look, *you* called *me,* okay? Don't act like a twat and waste my time, then act like I'm the one slowing you down.

She stormed away with a little waddle, stopped, and then called back to the driver, "Hey, can you pick me up from the hospital when the movie's over?"

I thought this would prompt another fight between the two, but the driver just sighed and said, "Yeah."

The patient climbed in the rig on her own and laid on the cot. She kept fidgeting during the ride and kept sticking her hand up the leg of her shorts and was trying to get the pickle out. Not even kidding, when we were about five minutes out from the ER, she managed to get this huge dill pickle out of her cavity.

She held it inches from my face and asked me, "Uh, what should I do with it?"

I jumped back so fast that I almost fell over. I was gagging when I pointed to the biohazard bin and yelled, "In there! Put it in there!"

What the hell did she think I was going to do with the pickle that just came out of her vagina, put it in a frickin' museum or something? Ugh. Gross!

She then asked, "Hey, can you drive me back to the movie, since I got it out?"

Uh, that's a huge 'hell to the no.'

The patient whined and moaned and even tried to get combative with us because we refused to transport her back to the drive-in movie area. When we got to the ER and tried to walk her inside, she attempted to run, lost one of her flip flops, and face-planted on the ambulance bay floor. So, she had to register in the ER anyway because she busted her lip open by acting like a jackass.

That was the weirdest call I've ever responded to, and I had to listen to my partner complain the rest of the night because he never did get that hot dog.

-T.E.

Location withheld at request

It Comes at Night

I work on the mental health unit and have been there for 10+ years. As you can imagine, our patients often present to us some off-the-wall stories.

My coworkers and I have heard it all, from one of our patients swearing to us that he was the reincarnate of Marilyn Monroe, to another patient becoming violent and requiring forcible restraints and sedation because she stated a demon was following her and body-jumping from person to person, and that she had to be the one to kill it (she violently attacked a few members of our staff and was eventually transferred to a live-in facility because she was in no condition to be released to family).

Sometimes, patients behave like the patient I will tell you about, by displaying childlike behavior. Mr. Smith, a 40-something-year-old, displayed childlike behavior of the following: he wanted to hold hands, threw tantrums when he couldn't play games or watch television, liked to draw and color with crayons, stated he couldn't eat unless his food was cut by a nurse, and, well, bedtime for Mr. Smith fits the bill for what you'd expect to deal with if you have a child. Mr. Smith, for example, cried when it was time for bed. He pulled out every excuse as to why he couldn't sleep. Each night, a staff member had to read him a story while he ate his nightly snack of pretzel sticks and cheese, tuck him in, and then deal with him getting out of bed four million times and screaming down the hall that he was thirsty, needed to use the restroom, or whatever excuse he had. Most nights, we'd have to react like angry parents to get him to get in bed and stay in bed, usually by threatening to 'ground' him from the next day's television time or tell him that he couldn't have dessert for a week.

Mr. Smith started behaving strangely. He'd scream bloody murder and would run out of his room, hollering about a rat in his room. When we'd go in there and turn on the lights, we couldn't find a rat, though Mr.

Smith repeatedly assured us it was there. After a few nights of this, he said he wanted to sleep with the lights on. For some reason, our Charge wouldn't allow this, so we bought Mr. Smith one of those cheap round nightlight things you can buy for, like, $1, so all he had to do was press the center of this light to have a nightlight.

It didn't help.

Mr. Smith was staying up all night out of fear and it got so bad that we had to force him to take meds to help him sleep because he was scared the rat would get him if he slept. If we let him stay up throughout the night, he'd behave like a cranky toddler during the next day, biting, kicking, and crying. He swore up and down, though, that he'd been attacked at night by this rat. We refused to entertain the nonsense, especially since we found absolutely no evidence of a single rat or any kind of infestation in Mr. Smith's room. We even put out no-kill traps under Mr. Smith's bed and in the corners of the rooms. For sure, if he had a rat sneaking in his room at night, it would wind up in one of those traps.

I'd say it had to have been about a week since Mr. Smith first complained of seeing the rat in his room that we noticed he had scratches and what appeared to be bites on his feet, arms, and hands. These were consistent with Mr. Smith's complaints over the week that he'd been attacked.

We presented photographic evidence of Mr. Smith's wounds to our Charge. She stated that Mr. Smith caused these wounds to himself and refused to allow us to use a video system to monitor Mr. Smith's room. Against her orders, we did it anyway, by using one of our tech's video baby monitors that linked a live video stream to her phone.

That night, we completed Mr. Smith's bedtime routine. I read him part of 'Cloudy with a Chance of Meatballs' while he snacked from his paper cup filled with pretzels and cheese cubes. He fussed a little when it was time for him to drink his medicine, but I finally got him tucked in and assured him that if a rat really was coming to visit him, we would know for sure. I explained the baby monitor setup to him. That seemed to calm him down a lot, but he begged for me to stay in his room, so the rat didn't hurt him again.

We waited and waited for the baby monitor to catch motion in the room, but after a few hours, there was still no alert. We started doing our charting and stuff and figured the Charge was correct.

I'd say it was about 03:30 when our tech's phone dinged.

She excitedly ran to her phone, pushed a button to monitor the feed, and gasped. I ran over to look at the screen.

"What is that?" I asked.

The face right-up in the camera of the baby monitor certainly resembled a rat, but as it moved around, I could tell it wasn't a rat. It had a long, slender body. It kind of looked like a weird snake with fur.

"That's a ferret, stupid," the tech teased.

"Huh?"

"A ferret. My sister has three of them."

"Are they like rats?" I asked.

The tech shook her head and said, "Uh, not really. Well, yeah, kinda. A lot of people keep them as pets. They're usually really nice if they're handled properly. They're really sneaky. My sister's, they used to be able to open their cage door, so she'd wake up the next morning and find her ferrets all over the house. One liked to get out and sleep on top of the cat tree with her cat."

We continued to watch the animal as it walked all over Mr. Smith's nightstand and ate leftover pretzels from his snack cup.

"That's what it wants," the tech said. "It's been coming in for his pretzels and crumbs."

The ferret snaked itself under Mr. Smith's blankets and we could see this lump moving around as Mr. Smith slept.

The tech went in the room and tried to catch the ferret, but she said it saw her and shimmied itself up between a pipe and the wall, before it escaped through a loose vent cover.

Mr. Smith woke up from the commotion and started crying. He refused to go back to bed, so we broke the rules again and let him bring his blanket and pillow to our station, where he slept on the floor. I do want to stress that we would never allow this with any patient if we thought he or she would behave in a violent manner against our staff. We felt comfortable with Mr. Smith in the way that he behaved like a child, and we could handle him (even when he lashed out) without additional staff.

We called maintenance right away and explained the problem.

"I'm telling you," the guy argued, "that there are no ferrets running around this hospital."

He set up a live-trap, anyway, and an hour later he had himself a ferret eating pretzels from behind the bars of a wire trap.

We're still not sure how the ferret managed to get in the building or the crawl space. We're not sure if it ever visited other units or patients. I do know that the hospital did contact the Humane Society, and volunteers took in this animal, which they couldn't determine if it was domesticated or wild by its behavior. After that, I have no idea what happened to the ferret.

The morning after the incident, we explained to Mr. Smith that the animal was not a rat. We lied and told him a sick person brought their pet to the hospital and that it escaped and visited him because it knew he had pretzels and it accidentally bit him in the night because it became scared when it was searching his bed for crumbs. Mr. Smith's response was to cry and say, "I hope that person isn't going to die." He seemed much happier when we informed him that the sick person was all better and that they were going home and taking the ferret with them.

Mr. Smith was eventually released to his sister's custody.

-I.J.

Wyoming

Ahoy

This is a story I made sure to tell my husband of 27 years, just in case he ever decided to stray. I'm going to tell the story in chronological order based on what we heard from LEOs, medics, the patient, the patient's girlfriend, and the patient's wife.

Jack and Jane Doe met at a club two months prior to the night in question. It was love at first sight. Jack was attracted to Jane's firm body and big breasts. Jane had allegedly been excited to learn that Jack, only a few months prior to the two meeting, had inherited a nice amount of money from a deceased relative. Allegedly, Jane had been particularly excited that Jack owned a very nice boat that he kept at the local marina. Jack and Jane had hot, wild sex on the boat the night they met, and that's apparently all it took for the two to become absolutely smitten with each other.

Within two weeks of meeting, Jack and Jane married in a courthouse ceremony.

Jack's friends thought he was crazy. Jane brought eight of her girlfriends to the courthouse to act as bridesmaids. For the ceremony, Jane wore a bikini and a knitted fishnet dress she found on Etsy for $14. As soon as they were officially married, the couple and their friends went to the beach, got hammered drunk, and Jane was arrested for fighting with a stranger because she swore Jack and the stranger were flirting. Jane's BFF bailed her out of jail, and Jane made up with Jack the next day by saying, "Baby, it just makes me crazy to think of some skank flirting with my husband."

Over the course of a week, Jane bought her way out of her apartment lease. She moved in with Jack. They went shopping and maxed out two of Jane's credit cards because she did not care for his home's décor. She decided that the house would seem more like a home if she could decorate with pink and purple throughout the residence. The two fought about this, but they eventually reconciled.

Two months after they married, Jane began suspecting Jack of having an affair.

Jack would allegedly come and go 'to work' at odd hours, even on his scheduled days off. Sometimes, he would smell of perfume, or he'd have lipstick residue on his clothes or skin. He had also been texting inappropriately to other females. He told Jane that the texts were innocent fun and that he'd never cheated on her and never would.

Jane did not believe Jack, especially when she realized Jack would display evidence of boating on a regular basis, even if he said he had to go to the office to work. Because she did not trust him, Jane took Jack's phone while he slept, and she installed a paid GPS app on it. She apparently hid the icon in a folder labeled 'Junk Stuff.'

One night, Jane observed Jack using his phone excessively. Jack then told Jane that he'd been called in for an after-hours meeting at work. Jane waited until Jack left, and she then used her phone to track Jack's location.

When the avatar representing Jack appeared on Jane's phone screen as being at the marina, Jane drove to the marina and stormed to Jack's boat.

Jane boarded the boat and found Jack having sex with one of the friends Jane had invited to their wedding to be a bridesmaid. At this point, everyone involved agreed that Jane was 'pretty mad.'

Heartbroken and irate, Jane took off one of her flip flops and threw it at her ex-friend, hitting the young woman in the face. The ex-friend attempted to push Jane off the boat, but as a fight ensued, Jane managed to reach the flare gun from the emergency bin that was kept on deck. Jane pointed the flare gun at her ex-friend.

Jack used this moment to tell Jane that it wasn't what she thought it was. Even though Jane caught the two in the act, Jack assured Jane that he and the ex-friend had never had sex.

Jack allegedly stated, "I didn't even put my dick in her. I was just dry humping. That's not cheating."

Jane, in a fit of rage, aimed the flare gun at Jack's genitals and informed him, "You can't cheat if you don't have a dick."

So, after Jane fired the flare directly at her husband's penis, she allowed her ex-friend to call 911. While they all waited for EMS and police to arrive, Jane started doing shots of 151-proof Everclear from the boat's bar.

When officers arrived at the marina and attempted to arrest Jane, she allegedly refused to cooperate with them. While she argued with them about their orders, she removed her top and bra. It was when EMS attempted to assess Jack's condition that Jane went even more off the deep end. She allegedly jumped on a medic's back and bit his ear so hard that she tore it. The medic's partner was able to remove Jane from the medic, and then an officer tased Jane. The ex-friend requested a lift to the hospital after she fell on the marina dock and twisted her ankle.

From this one call, our ER received the following: 1 male, human bite to ear; 1 female, medical clearance; 1 male, partially severed penis and burns of second and third-degree to inner thighs and groin; and 1 female, ankle injury.

Our medic patient required three sutures. The ex-friend was given a prescription for Motrin and was instructed on how to treat a sprained ankle. Jane was started on an IV and was transferred to ICU for the night because she was in and out of consciousness and had a BAC of more than .35.

Jack. Oh, my. Poor Jack. Let me tell you about Jack.

Jack's penis was mangled. It looked like he stuck his penis in a meat grinder, at least in some places. It was barely attached to his body. His burns? Phew.

Let's just say that the flare gun messed Jack up good. He was in such horrible shape that he could barely speak. We relied heavily on the injury to be explained by Jane's ex-friend. Jack received surgery.

According to the officers involved in this case, Jack told them that he cheated on Jane because they'd been married 'so long' that she decided she could 'let herself go.' He also allegedly stated that Jane wasn't 'putting out' as much, and that he knew her ex-friend would because [his] friend said that the ex-friend was easy.

I'm sure you have probably guessed by now that Jane was arrested for her actions against her husband. I'm not sure what happened to either, but I would hope that *someone* would file for divorce or annul it or *something*.

Now, I'd never do something like shoot my husband's penis off with a flare gun, but I think he thinks it's a bad thing that the option is now even in my mind, having seen this happen.

On another note, this didn't even make the news! You'd think something like this would be all over the media, but I never even saw so much as a tiny mention about it!

--G.R.
Florida

<u>Unbelievable</u>

Kerry, there is nothing funny about what I'm going to tell you, but if you have current EMS or healthcare professionals reading your books, I hope it gives them a jolt of reality and reminds them they should *always* properly document, even when they think, 'Oh, that won't matter later, anyway.'

Many, many years ago, before I retired from the local fire department, I witnessed a vehicular accident while I was on duty. In fact, I had been standing just outside the station, watering our plants, when I watched a box truck speed through an intersection and slam into a compact SUV that was rightfully driving through a green light. In the few moments it took me to process what I'd witnessed, 911 calls poured in and dispatch called our guys to the scene. EMS and police were on the way.

On scene, a male staggered out of the box truck. He seemed in okay shape, at least for going through an accident of that caliber. I instructed him to sit on the ground and wait for EMS. He did not comply.

I did not have time to babysit this man, as the SUV was in bad shape. The vehicle had flipped during the accident, and it was beat to all Holy Hell. At this point, I was deeply concerned about the vehicle's passenger(s). It was as I was trying to gain access to the vehicle that I noticed a sticker on one of the windows. That sticker had the names of the family and little characters to represent them, kind of like those stick figures. I could see from the sticker that it was a family of three: mom, dad, and a young female. This made me even more frantic as I attempted to gain access to the vehicle.

My worst fears were realized once I was able to pry one of the doors open. A female was in the passenger seat, and a young female who looked just like my granddaughter had been thrown from the back and landed in the front. I do not feel comfortable sharing details of this, but it was clear the child was deceased. I quickly felt for a pulse, anyway, even though I knew it would be almost impossible that she could still be alive, and even if she had shown signs of life, nobody could have saved her.

I scrambled to reach the adult female. As I was doing this, I radioed for a helicopter that was grounded not far from our location to be advised of the situation and be ready to fly. Unfortunately, the adult female was apneic and had no pulse. I could not remove her from the vehicle, as she was pinned. Because our station protocol calls for it, in situations such as this, when a patient shows no signs of life, we do *not* fly out to a trauma center. Instead, we continue rescue operations and EMS transports the patient to the nearest hospital.

I notified the helicopter crew that they could stand down, and I called in my findings to EMS, who arrived just a minute or two later. We worked to remove the adult from the vehicle, but she was pronounced dead shortly after EMS arrived.

During all this time, as you could imagine, I wasn't really paying that much attention the driver of the box truck. So, when officers arrived and couldn't find the driver, I didn't know what to tell them. It made me so mad to think that he could have purposely fled because he knew the severity of the accident and, undoubtedly, was at fault.

Officers found the driver one block over, after a complaint came in from a local bar. The driver was demanding alcohol, but the server felt the man was already too intoxicated or was under the influence of another substance. The driver was transported by officers to the local hospital, where a drug and alcohol test was administered. It was discovered that the driver was driving under the influence of both alcohol and illegal drugs when the accident had occurred. In our state, if a driver is found to be under the influence at the time of an accident where death has occurred, he or she is held liable for death(s) related to the accident, should any occur. So, not only was this driver looking at losing his job, (probably) his CDL, and being hit hard by insurance, but he was also looking at

DUI/DWI and criminal liability for two deaths.

I returned to the station and documented the scene and my actions to the best of my (shaken) ability. I said that I arrived on scene and witnessed a male exit the box truck. I said that the male did not appear to have life-threatening injuries, so I informed him to be seated until EMS arrived. I stated how I checked life signs of both females in the vehicle, and I stated that station protocol required medical transport of the individuals to the local hospital because they had no signs of life. I sent copies to everyone who needed them, and then I prepared myself to go home for the evening.

Right as I was walking out of the station, one of my guys hollered for me and said I had a phone call.

I listened as I was informed the driver of the SUV had been 25-weeks pregnant. This was not discovered until the patient's husband was notified and asked if they saved the baby. I physically felt ill and vomited into a trash can before I began crying and slinked down the wall. One of my guys had to finish the phone call and I couldn't drive myself home. Someone asked if I wanted my wife to come pick me up, but after witnessing that accident, all I could think in that moment was something like that happening to her. One of my guys gave me a ride home.

Honestly, I had absolutely no way of knowing this patient was pregnant. I did not see any physical signs that she had been pregnant, no pregnant belly, no vaginal bleeding that I could see on scene. Again, she had been pinned in the vehicle. But even when EMS and I removed her from the vehicle, I had no idea she was with child, none at all.

After telling some of my feelings to my wife, she suggested I seek counseling. I followed her advice and met with a counselor a few times over the course of a few months. Sometimes, I'd think I was 'fine' and had 'gotten over it,' but other times, I'd have a panic attack if my wife drove to the grocery store alone, or I'd find myself waking up in sweat, screaming. I was prescribed medication and continued with counseling until I learned coping mechanisms that I'd sworn for years that I didn't need to learn. My advice to anyone in the healthcare field is to utilize these counselors and any classes you may be offered. Even if you feel you have a handle on your emotions, please utilize these resources.

Time passed, and though the memories of that day became easier to deal with on an emotional level, they still lingered in my mind. Especially since it was so close to the station and there was now a memorial with wooden crosses, teddy bears, and flowers at the intersection, it was difficult to fully move on.

Somewhere in that time, I met with the patients' father and husband (the husband of the adult, father of the child). I tearfully recounted my actions. I showed him my report. I sobbed as I told him I had no inkling of an idea that she had been pregnant. We had a mediator present, just in case, but the husband/father said he held no malice towards me and he thanked me for responding to the scene so quickly. Some of my guilt and sorrow was lifted from my shoulders, but some was still there.

Five months went by. Six months. Eight months. A year. Seasons came, and seasons left. Mounds of snow became puddles that were swallowed by the ground and flowers grew. They tore down an old church that had been on the corner for about 85 years. Built a parking lot for a clothing store that's already gone out of business. The point is, life went on.

Almost two years following the accident, a well-dressed man in a nice car pulled up to the station as I was, again, outside watering the station's plants.

"I'm looking for a Mr. John Smith," he said to me.

I nodded and said, "You found him. How can I help you, sir?"

He extended a packet of papers and said, "You've been served."

I called our union attorney immediately. I was being named in a lawsuit. According to the papers, the driver of the box truck was being charged for three deaths: the female driver, her unborn child, and the young female passenger. His defense felt several things. Firstly, they felt the male driver was not liable for the unborn child's death because the child's mother should have been immediately flown to a trauma facility. The defense stated that, had I not notified the helicopter not to fly that patient, the child could have very well been delivered by a surgical team, and with the help of modern medicine, the baby could have lived. Therefore, the defense and their client felt *I* was the one criminally negligent in the case.

Secondly, the defense had obtained access to all first responder reports from the incident. They stated that nowhere in my report did I specify that their client climbed out of the *driver's side* of the box truck. Therefore, they felt that there was a discrepancy as to whether their client was even the driver, or if the driver of the box truck left the scene of the crime.

Additionally, the defense alleged that I did not offer proper care to their client, directly following the accident. They said I was under professional obligation to ensure their client was properly monitored, and because I neglected monitoring the patient to check on the patients in the SUV, their client, who was struggling with the demons of alcohol and drug dependency, was able to find his way to a bar. In fact, the defense stated that had I properly monitored their client, I would have noticed that he was the victim, that he was in shock. They insisted I was the reason the patient had tested positive for drugs and alcohol. I guess I should have had eyes in the back of my head to make sure this 'completely sober' guy didn't go off and score meth and liquor while the wife and daughter he hit lie dead in a mangled SUV. Shame on me.

I was found to be without liability in all charges, and the driver of the box truck pleaded down to avoid a longer prison sentence. He was sentenced to a year or so, I think. I heard that he could probably be out in a few months, if he could prove good behavior, enter a rehab program, and successfully prove to the court that he was remorseful of his crimes. It all sounded like bullshit to me. Do the crime, do the time is the way I see it. I don't know what happened to that man and quite frankly, I don't honestly give a rooster's crow because thinking about the heartache he caused and the possibility that he could have been walking around *months* after being sentenced to prison just really makes me irate.

I'm sorry that I couldn't tell you a funny story, I really am. I have a few from back in the day, but I felt this is the story I needed to share, because all first responders need to be positive to include *every little detail* in their reports, no matter how insignificant or obvious the detail may seem.

Since I retired, I have worked with the union as a speaker. I travel to different schools in the state and speak about fire safety. I also meet with firefighters all over to discuss the importance of seeking treatment after particularly difficult calls.

-Name and location withheld at request

Going Live

There are some sick people in the world but let me tell you about the sickest woman I've ever met in the 17 years I've been in nursing. The fact that she was so uncaring, and the absurdity of her actions still have me shaking my head.

Our ED received a toddler after he ingested cleaning products in his family's home. His mother called 911 and the child was rushed to our facility via EMS, with a police escort.

I do not feel that I can go into detail about the child's condition and treatment while he was admitted to our ED, but I feel I can inform you that this child was in critical condition while we were awaiting a flight transport for the child to be transferred to a pediatric facility.

After about 35 minutes of the child being admitted to our facility, the mother told her pre-teen daughter to go out to the car for something. I watched as the daughter returned to the patient's room with three huge plastic bags. I didn't know what was going on.

A few minutes later, I entered the room to check my patient's vitals. You would never believe what the mother was doing.

The mother had her daughter standing in the middle of the room, using a cell phone to record, while the mother was standing with her ill toddler in sight, holding up a pair of leggings and a matching top. She was having a LIVE SALE FOR HER LEGGINGS BUSINESS! Right there in her son's room, right there as he was on a machine that was essentially breathing for him, right there as doctors and nurses were coming and going.

"You can't do that in here," I snapped. I admit, I was probably a little ruder than our ED would have liked me to be, but for heaven's sake!

"But I have to," the mother replied. "I have a daily live stream of my inventory."

"Ma'am," I said, "I can not allow this, especially in the patient's condition."

I was especially careful with my words there, because I didn't want to say 'your son,' or say, 'with your son being in critical condition.' She gave me a gut feeling that she'd be the kind of person to try to sue the hospital for HIPAA.

The mother argued with me, and then the pre-teen daughter started in by calling me all kinds of names I would have never *dreamed* calling my parents. I tell you what, had I said even half of what that girl said to me to my own parents, I wouldn't be here to tell you this story! And if she were my daughter and dared saying anything like that to me, she'd be in the next room, having her teeth surgically replaced and getting the bar of soap dislodged from her throat.

A coworker heard all the screaming and called security. Thankfully, the woman and her daughter calmed down once guards arrived, but until the flight arrived, each time I'd enter the room the two would mumble under their breaths or complain loudly about how I was making them lose money. At one point, just as my gut told me, my patient's mother stated she was going to sue me for negatively affecting her income. I contacted the Nursing Supervisor, who had me write up a report for HR and Risk Management, just in case.

I'm not sure what happened with my patient. I hope he survived this incident. I do know that in any event like this, we notify Child Services, and they open a case to interview and/or monitor the child and any other children in the home. I'm not ill-willed; I hope the children are safe and happy. But, I also wish someone would smack that woman upside the head for her behavior while her son was admitted for an emergency.

-K.E.
Wisconsin

Hey, That Was a Good Idea!

We received a call of respiratory distress at an elementary school, involving a woman in her 30s. Dispatch stated the patient was having an asthma attack and did not have her albuterol inhaler. The patient's husband and other adults were nearby, attempting to keep the patient calm and instructed her to breathe, but she could not.

When we arrived, the patient had fallen unconscious and at the time was not breathing. School officials had enacted a live fire drill, but it was still in process when we arrived and young children were screaming and crying. We performed a brief round of CPR on the patient and administered oxygen once she was breathing on her own and was conscious.

The patient's husband, the entire time, kept apologizing and saying this was his fault.

This left me confused, really, and the only reason I could think he said that is because he possibly forgot his wife's inhaler, perhaps at home or something.

The patient requested medical transport, and she requested her husband accompany us. A family friend would drive to the hospital with the couple's young daughter after the child performed her role in the class play.

On the way to the hospital, we learned exactly what happened, and I was laughing so hard that my sides hurt for three days.

According to the couple, the wife couldn't get off work to get her daughter ready for the play. This meant that dear ole daddy was responsible for curling his child's hair, applying her face paint, and getting her in costume.

Well, maybe this would have been great, had a huge storm not just blown through the county, disrupting power all over the place. Our station was even running on generators, and we heard the ER was too. More than half of the county was without electricity.

Dad panicked. His wife had already stressed the importance of curling their daughter's hair because the child was supposed to be playing a lion, and it just 'wouldn't look right' to have a lion with straight, limp hair.

The girl's dad had an idea. He fired up his grill, took his daughter outside, and he heated the curling iron on the grill and then used it to curl her hair. He admitted to multitasking, and while he was waiting for the curling iron to heat up again, he began painting a nose and whiskers on his daughter's face. He then went to curl another section of his daughter's hair, but the curling iron was so hot that it burned the hair off.

Well, the dad took his daughter to the school auditorium, where her mom was waiting. Everything was fine and dandy, until the daughter spun around, and mom saw a huge bald spot on her child's head. This sent Mom into an asthma attack, and she panicked even more because she realized she'd left her inhaler at work and did not have a backup inhaler in her car.

The wife was still pretty angry as we drove to the hospital. The husband, at one point, looked to me and said, "Hey, that was a good idea?"

When I didn't immediately respond with anything but a 'maybe not, bud' look, he shrugged and said, "Whatever. I'm a genius."

-E.J.
Idaho

The Wheels on the Bus Go Round and Round

We responded to a call in what many would refer to as a 'bad' part of our inner city. Many of us have been ordered to never enter that part of town without a police escort, usually at night or if there's been a significant newsworthy story out of that part of town recently.

I must be the odd one out, because when I go over there, I hardly ever have beef with anyone. I think that's for several reasons. For starters, my grandmother lives in that neighborhood. (She's been burglarized three times, mugged twice, and has even been hospitalized, but she absolutely refuses to leave the area because that's where she and my granddaddy bought their first home and lived until he passed a few decades ago.) Secondly, you have to look at who I am as a person. I rarely argue with anyone or even acknowledge confrontational behavior. I find that helps me. Thirdly, and perhaps the most telling reason idiots leave me alone is my stature. I am 6'5", weigh 320-pounds, and I strength train so I can participate in strongman competitions. If you are unfamiliar with these completions, I basically go up against other strength trainers to lift weights and weighted objects in excess of 500-pounds. (As you can guess, everyone wants to be my partner, particularly on lift assists, ha ha.)

Well one day, we were called to a report of a fall. A woman stated her 83-year-old father missed a step on their basement stairs, and she requested medical transport. We parked street side and entered the residence. For 10 minutes, the patient argued with us and with his family, and it was finally decided that we drove all the way across town for nothing. The patient refused medical transport and said, "Damn kids think everything is an emergency." He held up one of his hands, which was missing two fingers and a thumb and said, "I didn't even go to the hospital when I did this! And I've lived 64 years!

You go to the hospital to die, and I ain't ready to die."

Fair enough, old man. Fair enough.

My partner exited the residence first and all I heard was, "Hey, what the hell are you doing?"

He sounded frantic, so I rushed outside and saw four males running away from our bus. The cab's passenger side door was wide open. We inspected the interior and found only a soft case filled with DVDs had been stolen. My partner was not too upset about that because they were DVDs he stole from a roommate who'd stopped paying rent and had to be forcibly evicted.

Okay, so we'd had our excitement for the day, so we hopped in the bus and started to go. Nothing seemed wrong or out of place.

Well, I hit 40 MPH in a 30 MPH zone and the entire front end of the bus started shaking.

"We're having a damn earthquake!" I yelled, as I tried to keep the bus straight and in my lane.

All of the sudden, no matter how hard I was yanking on that steering wheel, we veered into oncoming traffic, just barely missed hitting another car head-on, and we crashed into a telephone pole, which cracked and fell over halfway. My partner and I were shaken up, to say the least.

I radioed for help while my partner got out of to take pictures of the damage.

"Yo," he yelled, beating on my window like a psycho, "come see this."

I wrapped up the call with dispatch and got out to check out the damage, too.

It wasn't just a case of a bad, unexpected wreck. I can tell you that for damn sure.

The driver's side tire was almost completely off, and the brake rotor was sitting on what was left of the tire.

It didn't take long to figure out why this was. See, those guys we'd seen run off only minutes earlier, they'd tried to steal the tires off the bus. The cops and a tow truck came, and they said the tire that fell off was probably almost already off when we drove away. I

144

don't know how the hell I didn't notice the tire had been tampered with. Upon closer inspection, the cops and the tow truck guy saw that the back tire was loose, too, and it was missing lug rods.

Our bus went out of service, obviously, and my partner and I were assigned to another bus as soon as we got back to the station.

I know this happens to personal vehicles in many neighborhoods across the country, but I never thought anyone would be stupid enough to try it with EMS. And, I mean, think about your own grandmother or mama. Would you want your mama dying on the kitchen floor and we can't take her to the ER because someone screwed with her transport? Come on, now.

This is why we can't have nice things.

-C.W.
Michigan

I'll Go Crawl in a Hole Now

I don't know about you guys, but I'm the queen of embarrassing myself. I have done so many idiotic things that I don't even surprise myself anymore. I've closed my hair in my car door in front of a cute guy. I've almost knocked myself out walking into poles. Don't even get me started on how my brain forgets how to use basic reasoning when I'm nervous.

Luckily, readers have been kind enough to share some of their embarrassing moments. Here are a few:
∎∎∎∎∎∎∎∎∎∎∎∎∎∎∎∎∎∎∎∎∎∎∎∎∎∎∎∎∎∎∎∎∎∎∎∎

My boyfriend and I are both nurses. He works in Peds and I work in Cardiology.

I transferred one of my patients down to the ER following an emergency, and on the way back to the elevator, I saw my boyfriend walking ahead of me with another guy I knew from Peds.

146

I was trying to be playful, so I ran up there and squeezed his butt.

When he whipped his head around, I knew I made a grave mistake.

This guy wasn't my boyfriend! I mean, sure, he wore the same color of scrubs and seemed to have the same haircut. Then again, a close-shaved cut isn't really that uncommon, but I really thought I knew the back of my boyfriend's head better than that.

The tech accompanying this man introduced him as a physician visiting from a prestigious pediatric hospital. He was wearing hospital scrubs because someone spilled coffee on him an hour prior to me seeing him. It turns out, that person was my boyfriend. If that story doesn't tell you that we're made for each other, I don't know another one that will.

This visiting doctor laughed off my mistake. When the tech blabbed to the doctor that the coffee-spiller was my boyfriend, the doctor gave me a second look, said, "That explains a lot," and then walked away.

-H.C.

California
■■

I'm a housekeeper and was down at the ED, changing out trash cans and stuff, when I saw one of the girls at the counter was becoming frustrated. I could just tell by the way she was talking under her breath and slamming stuff around as she was trying to make copies.

A few seconds later, I heard the girl grunt, "You know, sir, it wouldn't kill you to talk to me and stop acting like you're too good."

I glanced up because I thought she was being incredibly rude, and I saw one of my neighbors.

"Hey," I said to the girl.

She ignored me.

"Hey," I said again. "I think you need some help."

"I'm busy right now," she said. "Apparently, all these old people think it's okay to complain about millennials, but here they are, standing in front of me and acting

148

like they don't have any manners. He won't even answer any of my questions. He just points at stuff."

My anger finally got the best of me, I'm ashamed to say. My sister is also hearing-impaired, and my parents always talked about how they decided to purchase my childhood home after meeting this neighbor. He comes to all our family cookouts and everything. It really bugged me that this girl was treating him like that. I threw down a bag of trash that was in my hand, walked over to the desk, and I screamed, "He's deaf, you moron!"

I signed to the patient, "I'm sorry, Mr. Smith. She didn't know you can't hear."

When I turned around, I saw the head nurse standing in the doorway with some paperwork. I thought she was going to tell me that she was going to report me and get me fired, so I was really worried because this is the only job I could find that had good pay and let me go to school during the day and take time off for school when I needed to.

Instead, she pointed and said, "I think he's trying to talk to you."

Mr. Smith wanted me to be his interpreter. He was having chest pains and didn't have time to wait around for the hospital to call in someone who could sign, and he was afraid writing everything down would take too long.

The girl at the desk was so embarrassed that she turned red and asked someone else to take over for her for a few minutes.

I never got in trouble. In fact, the hospital asked me if they could add me to a list for staff interpreters/translators and said any time they need an interpreter for ASL, they will see if I'm on shift or available. I get paid more now because of my ability to sign, so that's pretty cool.

-A.R.
Georgia

■■■■■■■■■■■■■■■■■■■■■■■■■■■■■■■■■■■■■■■

I have always had a habit of quietly singing or humming to myself when nervous.

My first stand-alone job where I didn't work under another physician was at a clinic in an inner-city. The clinic mostly saw homeless and low-income patients.

My first real patient came to the clinic with a complain of vaginal pain, so I had begun an examination. The patient was ungroomed and had pubic hair coming out of the legs of her panties.

As I was performing the examination, the patient started getting frustrated, and the nurse in the room kind of stared at me with a look that ordered, "Stop!"

"Was I hurting you?" I asked the patient.

"Why you singing that song?" she demanded.

It hit me, and I felt so bad.

I had been quietly singing 'Welcome to the Jungle.'

Oops.

-J.D., OB-GYN
New York

I was down at the ED registration area because there had been a situation with an angry family, and they wanted to speak to me, House Supervisor. I was trying to get the clerk's side of the story, but she had to run papers to the Charge, so I waited in the registration office for her return.

I saw a patient sitting in one of the chairs along the wall. The way that the area is set up, I could only see the top part of the man's body because the rest of him was obscured by the wall and glass window for the clerks.

The guy asked me where the elevators were, because he'd just been discharged from the ED and his friend was on Rehab.

"Feeling a bit lazy today?" I joked. I laughed and said, "I didn't feel like taking the stairs today, either."

The patient rolled his wheelchair out to where I could see that he only had one leg.

I tried to apologize, but he just shook his head and said, "You know what? I'll find someone else to help me."

I was mortified!

I actually went to my office and found some gift cards to a local restaurant and tracked the man down on Rehab. He was much more understanding when I explained that I'd been unable to see his condition and that I was just trying to make a joke. Still, I thought of that incident for weeks and cringed every time.

-S.K.-T.
Delaware
■■

It was 'breakfast for dinner' day in the cafeteria, and I knew I had to get down there because my very-pregnant wife (who also works at the hospital on another floor) craves the cafeteria's sausage. Even though I *swear* these are the same damn sausages you can get at the grocery store, my wife *swears* they're not. It's so bad that she buys extra sausages to snack on at home because the hospital wouldn't sell her uncooked sausages shipped from the distributor to heat up at home. The other night, she woke up in the middle of the night and started hormone-sobbing because she had forgotten to buy extra links that morning.

Well, I ordered an entire take-home box of the sausages for her. When I was leaving the cafeteria, I saw my wife sitting alone, facing the wall. I knew it was her by the ponytail and her red sweater.

I sneaked up behind her, wrapped my arms around her, and whispered, "I saved you a sausage for when you clock out."

Holy crap, I've never seen a woman move so fast!

This woman, who was clearly *not* my pregnant wife, started screaming in front of everybody about how I sexually harassed her and assaulted her.

I had to go down to HR and they called in a bunch of people because the woman I'd hugged demanded I be fired. She wouldn't hear me out, and every time I tried to talk or even apologize, she went berserk and yelled, "Fire him! He has no business working around women!"

The Dean of HR got fed up of the woman screaming and told her that if she couldn't calm down, he was going to send her out to the hall and conduct the interviews separately. He did not want to do that because of the sensitivity of the accusations, but it looked like it was going to boil down to that.

I had to explain my wife's cravings, open the Styrofoam box to show that I'm a maniac who just bought out an entire order of 24 maple sausage links, and *then* they called my wife down to speak to her because they thought I was lying.

When she walked in the room and saw us all sitting around a table, I'm not even kidding, she said, "John, what's going on? Oh my God, do you have sausage in that box?"

Seeing my wife react that way without being informed of the accusations against me made the woman relax a little. HR gave me a lecture about properly identifying people before I touch them. My wife and her online baby group thought it was hilarious.

■■

My coworker was waiting by the restroom door for her elderly patient. We were talking about this book I was reading. It was called, 'Nursing is My Cardio,' by this person named Kerry Hamm. I don't know if you've ever heard of it or not.

Anyway, my coworker said, "Bring it over here and let me see it."

I decided that walking 10 feet was just too much for me after the last three hours I'd had, so I decided to send the book to her via air express, meaning I threw your book across the room for my coworker to catch.

Well, right as I threw the book, the patient opened the restroom door and got clocked in the face. I rushed over to assist, and luckily all she had was a scratch on her cheek. She laughed the situation off and wasn't a bit upset, but I had to report myself because I'd injured a patient.

I was suspended for 10 days without pay and am on probation for 90 days.

I regret thinking that throwing the book would be a good idea. I never thought I'd have anything to send to you about my job, but I guess your book literally inspired this story.

-R.H.

Tennessee

∎∎∎∎∎∎∎∎∎∎∎∎∎∎∎∎∎∎∎∎∎∎∎∎∎∎∎∎∎∎∎∎∎∎∎∎∎

I was checking in this woman for a complaint of neuropathy. She was a frequent, so she just babbled on and on while I was getting her checked in.

"Some days," she said, "I think my arms would hurt less and my life would be better if I just chopped them off and ran around with no arms."

She must have seen that my eyes looked like silver dollars due to the fact that while she was saying that, another patient had walked up to the kiosk next to us.

This man, who was a double amputee from the shoulders, just kind of stared at the woman in front of me.

Well, she got so flustered that she tried to apologize and then passed gas right in the middle of her apology! There was no mistaking it, either. She just let one rip, and it was so loud that everyone turned to see where it came from.

Wow, what a rough day she was having!

-A.T.

Washington
■ ■

I'm a 911 dispatcher and my call went something like this:

Me: 911, what's your emergency?

Caller: I need help. I need help right now. My sister was trying to hang something, and she fell off the ladder. She's not moving.

Me: Okay. Honey, where is your mommy? Can you find your mommy or daddy and give them the phone?

Caller: (No response.)

Me: Sweetheart, is your mommy or daddy home?

Caller: What are you talking about? I'm 33-years-old!

Yikes! My bad. In my defense, this woman sounded like she was about six or seven!

-J.D.

Ohio
■■■■■■■■■■■■■■■■■■■■■■■■■■■■■■■■■■■■■■■

I volunteer at the hospital to escort visitors to various locations around the facility. Nobody should ever be on hospital grounds without a visitor pass, employee badge, or hospital bracelet, just due to security concerns we've had in the past.

I was having one of those days. I'd woken up late, forgot half of what I needed at home, locked my keys in my car right before my shift was supposed to start. You get it, I was having a rough day. I'd been up studying for my NREMT exam and my mind was mush.

Well, this couple came in, and I'd seen them a thousand times before. They always volunteered to sit with patients on hospice, whether to read to the patients or just talk to them.

"I haven't seen you guys for a while," I said cheerfully.

"Yeah," the man said, "we, uh, we lost our daughter last month."

I don't know what I was thinking, I really don't, but I asked, "Oh, man. Did you find her yet?"

His wife's eyes got real big and I knew she wanted to say something, but she didn't.

It hit me that the man meant their daughter had died and I gushed, "I am so sorry. I'm so sorry."

"It's okay, really," the man said. "And thank you."

As they were getting on the elevator, I heard the wife say to her husband, "What's wrong with her?!"

Her husband whispered back, "Maybe she's mentally handicapped."

I felt horrible all day!

-L.A.

Missouri
■■

A frequent flyer called the station because if we have a basic or someone available, we *sometimes* offer transport to and from doctor's appointment and/or medical appointments free of charge. This woman was notorious for waiting until the very last minute to try to get a ride, and during times we couldn't offer the taxi service, she'd become belligerent and abusive.

Now, I didn't *know-know* her on a personal level, but I bartend at the Moose on multiple nights throughout the week and every weekend, and bet your ass, that woman is always there, even though the Moose is a town over from where she lives. Amazingly, her medical appointments are in the same town that the Moose is in, but she can never seem to find a ride there.

"I need a ride," she'd told me that day. "My appointment is in thirty minutes."

"That's kind of short notice, Jane," I said. "It takes about ten to fifteen minutes to even go one way."

"I can't be late, either," she said, "so tell them to hurry up. I don't have all day."

"Jane, I've told you before, you really should call sooner for these-."

"If you was charging, you could say something," Jane yelled at me. "Till then, just keep your trap shut."

"I don't know if I have anyone, Jane. I'll have to check. You know, on short notices like this, you could probably call the ABC Taxi Service."

"They want money. I can't afford to pay for a ride."

"One minute," I said.

I thought I pressed the mute button, so I turned around and yelled, "Hey, is John back there?"

"I'm right here," John said, from the side of the room. "What is it?"

"Lame Jane needs another ride. Has an appointment in thirty minutes."

"Hell. She couldn't call sooner?"

"Probably hungover," I said with a laugh. "She can get to the bar five nights a week just fine and spend seventy-bucks a night on drinks, but she has to free-ride to appointments to the doctor and welfare because she won't pay for a real cab."

John laughed and tried to get out of taking Jane, but he was finally reminded that he had little choice in the matter.

When I went to take the phone off mute, I realized I'd just hit the button to connect with a second line. And since that line wasn't in use, the button basically did nothing, and Jane had heard everything.

I kind of felt bad for saying everything I said, but only because Jane had heard it and I had to listen to her scream at me for five minutes straight. She called my boss and complained, too. I was written up, but my supervisor said it was just a formality. He did tell me to watch my mouth and it was 'bad form' to talk about people, but I think he knew me enough to know that I generally *don't* talk about patients, but I did hold a particular annoyance with Jane.

Well, even though Jane swore up and down that she was going to stop using our free taxi, she continued calling for calls and cussing us out, until finally, our boss banned her from our service.

-P.H.

Pennsylvania

I went up front for my next triage patient and once-overed the paperwork. The name was one you'd associate with a female, and the complaint was rather silly, especially after all the serious complaints we'd been seeing that morning.

I called out the patient's first name and then turned to registration to rant, "What kind of idiot comes to the emergency room because they broke a fingernail? People like that really need to develop some common sense and stop wasting my time with bullshit like this. Stupid people, I swear!"

The entire time I was going on this rant, registration kept giving me this look like, 'Oh my gosh, stop!' I realized why about five seconds after I wrapped up my rant.

A man standing in the lobby had overheard everything I said. He stepped forward and identified himself as my patient. I have never been so embarrassed in my life, especially after I saw that his broken fingernail was a little bit more than that and his nail bed had become infected following an injury.

The patient filed a complaint and I was not only written up, but I was ordered to attend a training seminar on sensitivity in the workplace.

I don't normally behave that way, so it was especially embarrassing that I lost my cool and in front of the patient.

-T.M.
South Dakota

■■■■■■■■■■■■■■■■■■■■■■■■■■■■■■■■■■■■■■■

Feeling Hot, Hot, Hot

One day last year, I got home from work and had to go back within 10 minutes of being home because I hurt myself.

My coworker signed me in and asked, "How did you cut your stomach like that?"

I told her I tripped over my feet and fell into the corner of the kitchen counter. I told the doctor and all the ER nurses the same thing.

That wasn't exactly the whole truth.

I don't have central air at my house, so I have one of those standing air conditioning units that vent air through the window with plastic hoses.

The heat index was 112-degrees when I clocked out from my registration job, and I only live a few blocks away, so my car's a/c didn't cool me down as I drove home. Then, I had to carry a 50-lb. bag of dog food inside, while I was wearing my stupid uniform polo, hospital cardigan, and black pants, so when I got in the house, I was sweating half to death.

I found the easiest way to cool off was to stretch my shirt over the standing a/c vent, and then pull my head into my shirt like a turtle going in its shell, so that all the cold air would rush to my face and over my chest.

I forgot to take my glasses off, so when I popped my head out of my shirt, my glasses fogged up from how hot it was in the rest of the room. I couldn't see where I was going, so I tripped over the bag dog food and fell stomach-first against the corner of my kitchen counter. I had to get five stiches, and then I had to buy a new work polo because I ripped mine and it was covered in blood.

I saw your post on Twitter about doing this (and I was really happy to see it, too, because I thought I was the only person who ever did it), and I agree, it really cools you off.

But, make sure not to do what I did because you'll have to live with knowing how stupid you are.

I still haven't told my coworkers the truth. I think some of them read your books, so I'm sure it's gonna come out eventually.

-A.S.

North Carolina

America, F*@#, Yeah!

I have to tell you guys something shocking. In all the time I've been working on this series or the last, I have never received so many submissions directly following a holiday...until this year's 4th of July. I have no idea what they put in the water, but it seems like people have been going hog-wild. Here are a few holiday happenings to blow your mind:

··

If you ever get the wild idea to insert a bottle rocket in the tip of your penis, you'd better pray that it actually shoots out, rather than explode on site.

I would say that I don't know what would cause someone to try this, but the patient's BAC levels were through the roof.

One time I got drunk and tried to order McDonald's from a mailbox during my walk home, but even then, I wasn't drunk enough to us my penis as a firework launcher, so...

-H.E.

Location withheld at request

■■

Last year I arrested a man for an odd display of 'patriotism.' He painted his penis red, white, and blue.

I arrested him for exposing himself to female joggers in the park, but not before I deployed my taser and had to call for backup.

-L.C.

Louisiana

■■

My ETOH patient just quoted the entire motivational speech from the movie *Braveheart* at the top of his lungs and while standing on his cot.

When I told him to sit down and shut up, he shouted, "Isn't this America?"

He then vomited and almost fell off the bed.

He's now in restraints because he punched a cop.

-R.T.
Location withheld at request
■■

Last 4th of July, a patient told me he was stabbed following an argument revolving around a Toby Keith song.

This year, he came back with another stab wound and informed me he was stabbed after he called Captain America a 'pansy-ass pussy.'

I suggested my patient either lay off the alcohol-fueled debates or try to drink with a crowd that wouldn't try to disembowel him.

-M.F.
West Virginia
■■

Don't try to shoot fireworks out of your butthole.

There, consider that a public service announcement.

You don't even want to know how many complaints of buttocks injuries I've seen this week.

-C.S., M.D.

Texas

■■■

"This is the land of the free!" my patient screamed, right before he was tased.

Well, not in my ED, when you've gone on a cocaine-induced rampage and flipped the crash cart that took me 20 minutes to stock, buddy.

-T.C.

Arizona

■■■

I feel that I shouldn't have to tell anyone not to light a firecracker and then drop it in your underwear, but apparently it needs to be said.

Severe burns to the genitalia. Transferred to a facility with a burn unit. I don't even want to think about what that bill is going to look like.

-N.O.
Arkansas
■■■

Summary of my last patient: PT complains of severe burns to calves and shins. PT states he and his brother consumed approx. 24 beers each and then played what he describes as 'fireworks baseball.' PT states he lit fireworks and pitched them to his brother, who would then attempt to hit them. PT states brother hit one directly at him and it exploded against his legs. PT believes event occurred one hour before he notified EMS. PT bases his timeline on amount of alcohol he consumed following incident.

-G.N.

South Carolina
■■■■■■■■■■■■■■■■■■■■■■■■■■■■■■■■■■■■■■■

When we arrived on scene, my patient was passed out on the sidewalk, wearing a latex Uncle Sam mask and a star-spangled speedo.

-H.D.

Washington
■■■■■■■■■■■■■■■■■■■■■■■■■■■■■■■■■■■■■■■

911 call, as told by G.P. from Florida:

Me: 911, what's your emergency?

Caller: My friend just ran inside and said my boyfriend shot himself.

Me: He shot himself?

Someone in the background: *laughing* Oh my God, did you see that? *laughing*

Caller: It's not funny, John. Go check on him. You have to make sure he's okay. Hurry.

John: He's fine. He shotgunned a 6 pack, so he probably didn't even feel it.

Caller: John, go check on him!

John: I already did. He passed out. *laughing* He's just laying out there.

Me: Ma'am, I need your location to send help.

Caller: *apparently goes to the back yard and screams directly in my ear* He's ruining the beer pool! Oh my God.

Me: Ma'am, I need your location.

Someone in the background: Man, you should've seen his face when that bullet hit him. Oh, man. Best 4th of July ever.

Me: Ma'am, I NEED YOUR LOCATION.

Caller: Oh my God. Is he going to lose his foot? There's blood everywhere. Is he going to die? He told me we're going to the concert next week!

Me: Ma'am-

Caller: Why aren't you doing anything? Why aren't you telling someone to help him?!

Me: Ma'am, please stay calm. I need your location.

Caller: What's the address here?

Someone in background: I don't know. I don't even know whose house this is. Jack just texted me and said to come to the party.

Caller: *screaming* Someone give me the freaking address! *mutters* Oh my God. You guys can find me when I leave from house arrest, but you can't send a freaking ambulance.

Medics found the patient with both legs in a plastic kiddie pool of half-melted ice and floating cans of beer, with his torso on the lawn. The patient was transported to the ER for a through and through GSW to the foot and was expected to make a full recovery.

It turns out, the partygoers had crashed at a stranger's home. The homeowner returned from a shopping trip while officers were taking reports, and five college kids were arrested.

▪▪▪▪▪▪▪▪▪▪▪▪▪▪▪▪▪▪▪▪▪▪▪▪▪▪▪▪▪▪▪▪▪▪▪▪▪▪▪

If you must remove any type of nest or hive from your property, I recommend calling a professional, rather than doing what my patient did.

This genius went out and shot a roman candle at a hornet's nest. He shattered the nest and was stung approximately 200 times, which landed him in ICU for observation.

Needless to say, my patient will probably not be in any sort of condition to attend our town's annual fireworks or attend any cookouts for the holiday.

During the time he was in ES, he told me that he regretted doing it, but 'it looked really cool.'

Maybe it did, but now my patient is covered in welts and I'm pretty sure his bill easily surpassed the $10,000 range.

-K.E.

Illinois
■■

We received a patient complaining of blood in her stool.

I was in the room as she was disrobing, and I saw a large bruise on her stomach. I didn't feel right asking the patient about it since I'm a tech, so I notified the patient's nurse. I thought maybe the patient had been a victim of domestic violence.

I've never felt more stupid in my life.

The patient sustained those contusions by doing a belly flop off the high-dive at the city pool.

She had blood in her stool because she sustained acute abdominal trauma from hitting the water too hard.

-K.W.

Iowa

■■

I just had to explain to this college girl that no, that was not blood in her stool.

Her loose stool was red because she took 14 cherry vodka Jell-O shots the night before.

-R.W., M.D.

I just adopted a large dog, and I thought it would be fun to take him to the park to get him used to people and loud noises.

Someone started setting off firecrackers, and the dog bolted. His leash got wrapped around my leg, and now I'm at work being treated for a dislocated knee. He's in the lounge with someone from Lab.

I've never had a dog before, so I really didn't think about him being scared of fireworks.

Now I feel like a bad dog owner and a bad coworker because I added to the chaos of the holiday.

-M.G.
Rhode Island

Badass Biker

We were running on generators because it had been storming all night. Our phones were out, so security went around the hospital and gave each department head a radio to contact other departments. Trust me, you don't ever, ever want to rely on a radio to relay an order to CS or find an ICU bed for your patient when you're swamped with patients. We had so many people trying to use their radios at once that the busiest departments made the tough decision to work short-staffed by sending one employee to the other department that had been attempting to contact the most. We had a CS employee and an ICU tech down in the ER, each writing down orders and requests, then they'd have to run all the way back to their respective departments, fill the orders or approve the requests, before coming back to the ER.

I am a tech and am responsible for registration, and I was finding it damn near impossible to keep up. I was drenched in sweat, my hair was a disaster, and I had cried three times in two hours, so I had black lines all over my face from where my eyeliner and mascara had run. Everyone was yelling at each other, and I felt like I was going to have a heart attack.

When this woman staggered inside, I knew it was serious. I mean, whenever there's someone clutching at a knife sticking out of their chest, I think it's safe to assume it's a serious situation. I grabbed gloves and dialed for help. Nobody answered.

I told the woman to stop, but she kept walking. There was blood dripping all over the place. The knife had gone through part of her leather vest, a tank top she was wearing under the vest, and was jutting out from above her left breast. She had blood on her hands, all over her torn jeans, on her leather biker boots, and even in her hair. Thunder rolled, and lightning cracked outside. I don't know why, but I imagined the woman fighting crime in the storm, kind of like a superhero in a dramatic cinematic scene. I'm sure it couldn't have been farther from the truth, but it was my escape for about 10 seconds.

"We're gonna get you some help," I assured her. "I have to find a bed for you first, but we're gonna get you help."

After a minute or so of arguing, the woman finally sat in a wheelchair. On my sixth call to the unit clerk and Charge, someone answered the phone and told me to get the patient back to a trauma room that had just been cleaned.

More patients were lining up in the lobby and they seemed impatient.

"Is anyone here bleeding or experiencing heart symptoms?" I yelled, as I walked around the lobby to the stab victim.

Everyone shook their heads. One guy said, "I haven't pooped in three days."

"You'll live," I said. "Just have a seat, and I'll be back up here as soon as I possibly can, okay?"

"Don't worry," I said to the stab victim. "I'm taking you back now, and they'll take real good care of you."

She gripped my hand and told me, "I need you to go out to the truck and get my husband. It's a big truck with a skull painted on the side. You can't miss it. I don't want him to be alone."

This woman begged and pleaded with me to get her husband that Charge sighed and ordered me to go find the man. I was pissed about it, too, because it was pouring outside, and I didn't know what kind of person I'd be dealing with since his wife had just been stabbed. Going to anyone's vehicle in the middle of the night is dangerous, and I didn't feel like it was my responsibility to do anything like that. I knew security was busy, though, because quite a few of our systems haven't been worked up to run on generator, so some of the alarms didn't work and certain areas needed to be monitored.

I put on a huge lab coat someone left on a chair and I rolled my pants to my knees. All the patients waiting to be registered gave me weird looks when I was walking through the lobby. I told them I'd be right back, and then I went outside.

The rain was really cold, but it felt good because I was so hot from running non-stop. The lab coat turned out to be a dumb idea because it wasn't keeping my scrubs as dry as I thought it would.

I looked around for the patient's truck and saw it. Of course, it was parked at the very far end of the lot, so I had to literally wade through ankle-deep puddles in the low parts of the lot. My shoes and socks were soaked by the time I got to the driver's side door.

I saw a big, burly man sitting in the passenger seat, curled up like a child, and he was crying. It was really strange for me to see because this wasn't a guy you'd pass on the street and think, 'Yeah, he's a crybaby for sure.' He looked like the kind of guy you'd pass and think, 'I bet he's been to prison at least twice.'

I knocked on the driver's side window and he appeared startled. It took a second, but he reached over and rolled the window down.

"Your wife wants you with her in the ER," I told him.

Right at that moment, lightning shot across the sky and the man screamed. He shook his head and told me that he couldn't go inside because he didn't want to be struck by lightning as he was crossing through the parking lot.

Bizarre.

I tried to coax the man inside for a minute or two, but then I went back inside, soaking wet, and had to inform his wife of what he'd said.

You would think that would be that, but she got out of bed as a doctor was assessing her wound, and she said she'd go get him herself. When staff basically told the woman she needed to sit down and get that knife out of her so she could be sutured, she went crazy and started threatening everyone. One of the nurses decided that it wasn't worth the drama, so she took an umbrella and went to the truck.

Ten minutes later, as I was standing in my sopping scrubs at the registration kiosk, I saw the nurse assisting the patient's husband inside. He was crying when he entered the lobby, and everyone was looking.

The patient had some complications from her wound and ended up being transferred to surgery. I don't think her husband ever left the waiting room.

I just thought I'd tell you about that situation because it was really weird, and the more I think about it, it's pretty funny to know that these two could get in a situation that involves stabbing, but the guy couldn't walk across the parking lot in a thunderstorm.

-J.W.
Oklahoma

Family Fun Day

Our hospital was hosting our annual Family Fun Day at a local amusement park, so the home was closed to general admission. Employees and their families had to present a special ticket to get in the gates, and from there, food and drinks would be available at discounted prices, rides would be free (and unlimited), and I think the only thing anyone would have to pay full-price for was to play the games or buy souvenirs. We'd hosted this event every year for more than a decade, and until the point in the story, we've never really had a problem.

On the day in question, it was already 90-something degrees at 08:00, so we were in for a long, hot day. Families were pouring in through the park gates, and I was in charge of taking photographs for our monthly newsletter, so I was just kind of walking around the park and doing my job.

Well, everything seemed fine until the temperatures soared to over 100-degrees. Then, I started seeing park security out and about a little more, and I started noting that every few minutes, I'd be hearing kids throwing temper tantrums or parents yelling. Surely, I thought, it was the heat causing these people to grow irritated and lash out.

Before I knew it, a group of pre-teens and teens rushed by me and attempted to grab my camera by its strap. I hung on because it's a $3,000 camera, and by hanging on while one young man pulled and ran, I felt my shoulder pop and the pain dropped me to the ground.

Realizing they weren't getting the camera from me, the kids immediately ran ahead and began bullying a small child in front of her parents. They ripped an inflatable game prize from her arms and popped it, kicked over the stroller with the child still in it, and when the father lost his temper, three of the older kids jumped him and started hitting and kicking him while his wife screamed for help.

While this was going on, some of the other kids ran and began ransacking the game booths. Helpless attendants stood nearby as these kids yanked stuffed animals and those little square framed posters from pegboards and carelessly tossed them to the asphalt walkway. In a matter of seconds, some of the booths were partially dismantled.

I couldn't believe my eyes.

Now, even with my shoulder pain, I knew someone, somewhere would need proof of the damage these kids were doing, so I started snapping away. I can't explain how unbearable the pain was because I later learned my shoulder was dislocated and a tendon had snapped, which required surgery. The pain was worse for me than childbirth was, but maybe because I didn't have any drugs to help me through the injury.

As much as adults were trying to subdue these kids, they were also fighting with each other. I'm not exactly sure how it came about, but I know one fight happened when I woman saw a man grab one of the teens by the arm and the woman screamed, "What is wrong with you? Spanking is the reason this kid is like this, in the first place!"

The man yelled back, "Lady, I'm just getting him under control. And, if he'd gotten his ass beat by his parents, I can guarantee he wouldn't be doing what he's doing."

The woman then pepper-sprayed the man for 'being violent.' It would have been one thing if she sprayed him once, but she had her finger on the nozzle release and was sending a constant stream of pepper spray at the man as he screamed and rolled around on the ground.

Now, another man witnessed this and attempted to take the pepper spray from the woman. She then turned the pepper spray on him.

Well, her husband walked up and thought she was being assaulted or something, so he started wailing on the guy who'd tried to take the pepper spray from the woman. Other people saw a fight and joined in. I guess it was for the sake of fighting, because at this point it didn't seem easy to discern why anyone was fighting.

Some of the older kids continued on their rampage, and all around me there was fighting. I watched as one man attempted to climb an antique Ferris wheel. Park Security couldn't get the man to come down, but I guess they didn't have to in the long run because he lost his grip and fell about 15 feet. (Don't worry, I heard he was fine.)

I was right in the middle of the riots you see on TV, and it felt like one, especially when someone set one of the trash bins on fire and that fire had spread to a souvenir shop.

Law enforcement was called, along with multiple EMS and FD units. It still took officials two *hours* to get everyone control. I can tell you that more than 10 people were arrested, and even more were transported to the nearest emergency room. There are still lawsuits going on today, and it's been a great deal of time since this has passed.

It has since been determined that several parents used the amusement park as a babysitter for their kids, and I think the cops said only one of the troublemakers had his parents at the park. The rest of the kids were dropped off by their parents and just felt like causing trouble, I guess.

Needless to say, the hospital's contract with the amusement park was canceled and the hospital ended up paying restitution to the park in excess of $10,000.

I can tell you this much: This is the closest I've ever been to believing that society is doomed. The way I saw all those adults turning on each other, the violence I witnessed... I simply don't understand how we've ended up here. I don't understand how we've seem to value disrespect and violence over compassion and peace. I guess that's a thought for another day.

Since I was on clock, the hospital paid for my injury, including time off and the physical therapy required for a complete recovery. I guess there's that, but I'm still shaking my head over what occurred that day.

-Name and location withheld at request

Listen to the Music

I received a new partner and didn't know if I was going to like her.

Our first run together was responding to an injured man at a bustling intersection.

When we arrived, the patient stood out like a hooker in Sunday school because he was the only one missing half his clothes and with a face covered in blood from a gash across his forehead.

Judging by the way this man was waving his arms and lunging at passing cars, it was clear he was under the influence. It would not be safe for my partner or me to attempt to reason with or treat the patient. Instead, we called for LEO assistance and waited in the rig.

At one point, after the patient removed his shorts and urinated on a bicycle that was chained to the front of a store, the man plopped down in the center of the sidewalk, sprawled out, and looked like he was going to take a nap.

My partner, out of dead silence and after us not speaking at all except to say 'hi,' when we were introduced, reached in her pocket and pulled out her phone. She tapped a button, looked at me, and looked at the patient right before I heard music and someone singing, "If I lay here… If I just lay here…"

I saw her Snow Patrol and raised by playing Queen's 'Sleeping on the Sidewalk.'

And that's how I knew she was going to be my favorite partner ever.

-D.F.
Indiana

The Test

This is a good example of a test you can perform to measure the length of time a person has been in the first responder field. Simply review the story, and then view the responses to know if you're dealing with a rookie or an old-timer.

At approximately 19:00 on a weekend, officers were called to Wal Mart for a report of four subjects shoplifting. They had loaded two push lawn mowers, a hot tub, live plants, various lawn and garden supplies, and power tools in a Ford Crown Victoria. Bystanders made a citizen's arrest on the vehicle's driver, who claimed he was asked by the subjects to drive them to the store. He claimed he hated Wal Mart, so he decided to wait in his vehicle until his passengers returned.

Officers arrived and were able to apprehend three of the subjects. A male fled on foot and officers chased him through the busy parking lot, but they lost him due to traffic. The male subject then crossed a four-lane highway, where he attempted to gain access to vehicles in a gas station parking lot. Upon realizing he could not gain access to the vehicles there, and upon realizing officers were closing in on his location, he fled again. This time, he ran to a nearby semi fueling station.

The subject found a parked semi that had a running engine. He attempted to steal the semi, but its driver (who'd been in the restroom), managed to climb up and yank the subject from the cab. The subject sustained a head injury as a result of this action.

Officers called EMS and while they awaited EMS response, they attempted to arrest the subject. The subject then reacted violently and pulled a weapon from his pocket. Because officers could not subdue the subject safely (for bystanders, officers, and the subject), a taser was deployed. It was reported that the subject urinated once struck by the taser.

EMS transported the subject to a local emergency room for a medical clearance.

Officers arrested the other three shoplifters and transported them to jail. The driver was released from the scene because officers believed his version of events and he was compliant. Officers worked with store management to return stolen items.

Take a look at the responses below to know what level of first responder you're dealing with.

Fresh-off-the-boat: "HOLY CRAP! Did you see that? Guys, seriously, did you see that? That's the wildest thing I've ever seen! I bet nobody can top that. There was so much blood! He was near death! I don't know why the cops tased, him, though. Maybe they need training, because all they have to do is tell someone to do something, and that person will do it."

Also acceptable: "This is the craziest day ever!"

The In-Betweener, who's been around long enough to have witnessed some crazy crap, but still gets worked up over certain things: "Damn, that was kind of crazy. I knew he was gonna run. Too bad I missed him getting tased."

Also acceptable: "That was a lot of blood, but the guy's fine. He'll have a lot to think about in jail."

The Veteran: "They sell hot tubs at Wal Mart?!"

Also acceptable: "The guy could drive a semi?" "All that stuff could fit in a Crown Victoria?"

Also acceptable: "Okay, pay up. I won the bet that he was gonna get tased." "I guess you could say he got the piss shocked out of him! HAHAHAHA."

<u>OMG, What?!</u>

A male Lab tech left my patient's room looking as pale as a ghost and gagging. I didn't know what to think because my patient was a well-groomed woman in her 20s, had no body odor that I could detect, and she wasn't wearing perfume that I knew of. She was in for something like dizziness, so nothing too severe.

"John," I called to him, as I raced to check on his condition, "what's the matter?"

He raised his arm halfway and weakly pointed to my patient's room. He said, "She just became the most disgusting point of my career."

I knew something major must have happened in that room because John's been in Lab for more than 30 years.

"Oh no," I said. "What happened?"

John tried to explain, but he became sick to his stomach and had to excuse himself. It was probably for the best because the patient's boyfriend exited the room to complain to me about John.

"My girlfriend's in there crying because of him," the boyfriend said. "She asked him not to use a needle, but he did it anyway."

I kind of offered a little shrug. It wasn't an 'I don't care' shrug as much as it was a, 'There were no alternatives' shrug.

"Sorry," I said to him, "but we haven't invented a sure-fire way to draw blood from a patient without using a needle. John is very good at what he does, so I'm sure he made it as quick and painless as possible."

"She told him to take her tampon. He could have done that."

I yanked my head up so fast to look at this guy's face that I swore I gave myself whiplash.

"She what?" I exclaimed.

"She told him to take her tampon. You know, so he could use it to find out what's wrong with her."

I had no idea what to even say back to that. I basically avoided the topic for as long as I could and just explained to the patient and her boyfriend that John needed to take blood from a vein.

I can absolutely see why John was so shaken up over the encounter, because even I was confused and shocked.

-K.I.

Mississippi

<u>Coming to America</u>

At the time, I was fresh out of nursing school. I had worked at a very tame, boring LTC (long term care) facility for a while as a tech and a gopher before I landed an RN position in the emergency room at one of our city's hospitals.

I quickly learned our Florida ER was the busiest, and especially on my shift, where I'd work 11A to 11P. As a new ER nurse, I was feeling completely overwhelmed by the fast-paced, chaotic environment. I barely made it through my first month. I'd be crying in the parking lot after my shifts, then I'd go home and cry myself to sleep. I didn't know how I was going to ever be as good as my fellow RNs, and I'd already seen so many tragedies that I found myself awake at 02:00, Googling how to cope with the stresses of caring for difficult patients or worse, losing a patient.

It's going to sound like I'm blaming you, but please know that I'm not. See, when I was in nursing school, I started reading your books. I cried at the sad stories and knew to expect them, especially in an emergency setting. Reading your books kind of helped me choose the ER as a place of employment because I wanted the adrenaline rush, and I wanted to help people when they needed it the most. But I guess I expected to see more stupidity come through the doors, as opposed to tragedy. I didn't want tragedy. I wanted one of the patients that you wrote about, at least just once. I couldn't take the seriousness for one more minute, but I didn't have much of a choice.

One night, I helped with a pediatric code. We all know codes are bad, but when the codes are kids, it's the worst thing in the world. My patient was 13-months-old. His mother and father were going through a divorce, and his mother told us that she'd petitioned the courts to either revoke the father's visitation or ask the courts to order supervised visitation. The courts denied her requests, so now she was standing in the lobby, not knowing that her son had died at the hands of his abusive father.

It was right when that patient's mother was informed of her son's death, right when she screamed loud enough that they could hear her in the cafeteria across the hospital, that I thought about throwing in the towel. If all my patients were going to be abuse victims or overdoses or MVA victims, I didn't know that I could handle that.

I asked Charge if I could take my lunch break early. She said no, that I had a patient out front. I had wells of tears in my eyes so thick that I couldn't see straight as I was going up front to call my next patient, who was probably a junkie looking for another fix.

I blinked away my tears and took a look at the patient queue on the triage computer. It was a male's name, I thought, and it was a foreign name. I did my very best to pronounce it correctly, but I'm sure I butchered it. The chief complaint entered by registration was 'buttocks problem.'

'Now, what the hell does 'buttocks problem' mean?' I thought to myself, as I waited for the patient to emerge from the waiting room. I tried to ask one of the registration clerks, but they were all busy.

My patient walked out of the waiting room and he was walking with his butt cheeks clenched together, doing kind of a short, slow waddle. Both of his hands were on his buttocks, like he had to hold his ass on to keep it from falling off as he walked. I started to think that maybe he had something stuck up there. That would sure be what I needed to get away from all the bad things I'd seen so far.

"Mr. Doe," I asked, as soon as we got to a room, "what's going on tonight?"

He waved his hands in front of his chest and shook his head.

"You can tell me," I said. "Don't be embarrassed."

"No English," he stuttered. "No English."

He then turned sideways and pointed at his butt.

"Need doctor," he said. "Doctor."

It took 20 minutes and four different interpreters from the hotline to figure out that my patient spoke a specific Russian dialect. From there, it was a lot easier, but weirder, too.

The interpreter translated my name and title to Mr. Doe. She translated when I asked why he was seeking medical treatment.

Mr. Doe then frantically started explaining, and at one point, he was even crying.

"Did you catch all of that?" I asked the interpreter.

She wasn't speaking, and I couldn't hear her on the line. I started to think that we'd somehow lost the connection, and I could feel an anxiety attack coming on. I started to take deep, calculated breaths.

"Uh," the interpreter finally said, "one second."

She asked Mr. Doe a question and he repeated what he'd just said. This time, he raised his voice and paced in front of the speaker phone.

"Nurse?" the interpreter asked.

"I'm here," I said.

"Um, the patient states that his anus is leaking."

"His what is what?" I asked, shooting a look of confusion at the speaker.

"His anus is leaking."

"Uh, okay…"

"He also wants to speak to a male physician. He says that it is inappropriate to be treated for this matter by a female physician."

"But his anus is leaking?" I asked. "Did he tell you anything more specific?"

"No," the interpreter replied.

I asked, "Well, can you ask him to please elaborate? Once I understand his concerns, I can request a male physician for further examination."

As the interpreter spoke to Mr. Doe, he became agitated and started saying, "No, no, no."

I don't know what the interpreter said to finally get him to calm down, but he sighed and started calmly speaking to her.

"The patient states that he was walking down the street, when he felt a tickle between his buttocks," said the interpreter.

The interpreter started to snicker, but she caught herself and managed a quick save by clearing her throat.

"He stated that he walked for two blocks before he could find a restroom," she continued. "It was there that he wiped a mostly-clear liquid from between his buttocks and groin area."

"Okay," I said.

"The patient says that he cleaned himself up, but as he continued walking, he could feel the tickle again. He returned to his hotel room and became worried of his condition. He also does not know how he will pay his bill, as he is unsure if his company will cover the costs. He is on a work trip to the United States."

"Please tell him a clerk will get that information after he's been discharged," I responded. "And please tell the patient that I will return with a male physician."

I didn't really have much to go on as I approached our only male physician. I explained what I had learned from the interpreter, explained that the patient wished to see a male physician, and then I was told to wait outside the room while the doctor went in to perform an exam.

Leaning up against the brick wall, watching all the hustle around me, I can't explain how I felt. In a way, I felt like a child, that the doctor wanted me to essentially stay where he could see me. In another way, I felt guilty because everyone else had a million things to do at once, and there I was, basically twiddling my thumbs while my patient was having his ass looked at.

A few minutes later, the doctor came out of the room. He was laughing so hard that his face was beet red.

He patted me on the shoulder and said after a few moments used for catching his breath, "Go in there and wrap up that call with the translator."

"But what's going on?" I asked.

"I just had to explain to our patient that he has the very-common American problem known as 'swamp ass,'" the doctor answered. "Explain discharge to the translator, and then get our guy out of here."

I knocked and entered. My patient was just pulling up his slacks and appeared embarrassed. He started speaking but wouldn't look at me.

"Operator?" I asked.

"Still here," she replied.

"Did you understand anything the patient just said?" I asked.

She laughed. She flat-out laughed and then said, "He said, 'It appears I have overreacted regarding this matter, and for that I apologize.'"

I started to explain the discharge process to the patient, but he must have interrupted me four or five times to apologize and speak in surprise that he received a 'swamp ass' diagnosis. (Just to clarify, our doctor didn't *really* use that term. The patient was given a diagnosis of 'unventilated perspiration.')

It took another 15 minutes to get through all that, but I was finally able to discharge the patient, and we transferred the interpreter to a registration clerk to assist the patient with the process of gathering his personal and insurance information.

The second my patient left the exam room, I literally sat on the floor and cried—but this time, I was crying because I was laughing so hard.

And that, I swear, was the best I'd felt in a long time.

That one confused patient really reminded me that everything *was* going to be okay. I know my story doesn't seem like much when you compare it to yours or the stories other readers have submitted, but it was kind of a big deal for me because I went from wanting to quit my job and go back to being a tech with a mountain of student loan debt, to wanting to hang in there and see what else the ER gods had to offer. It reminded me to step back, laugh a little, and try not to let my mind replay the tragedies on a loop. It helped me realize that I don't have to hold all that sadness and anger inside. It's okay to react to a situation, but it's not healthy to dwell on it. I needed this patient more than anyone could have ever known.

In a few days, I'll have been an ER RN for a year. I've learned how to control my emotions a little better, but I still have days/nights that I really do question everything about the world and about myself. Unfortunately, we still don't see a lot of silly things, at least not at a frequency I'd like, when compared with all the bad stuff we see. I think that's a good thing, though, because we just might have the only ER in the entire universe where patients actually come in for *emergencies*!

-J.M.
Florida

Look at That

A couple of years ago, a woman brought her boyfriend in because while they were at the lake, he set off fireworks in his hand and blew off two of his fingers.

Now, when the guy came in, he was so drunk that he could hardly stand on his own. I wouldn't have known, just looking at him, that he blew off any body part because he was so calm and collected.

Sure enough, though, two of his fingers were gone, so we transferred him to a trauma facility.

That part of the story wasn't so eventful, but this is where it gets kind of crazy.

I was also working the next day, and I remember being pretty angry about it because I clocked out at 02:00, had an hour drive home, and I was expected to be back at work at 07:00 for a 12. Screw employees needing to sleep or unwind from a job where people die in their arms, right?!

215

Anyway, I was hiding from Charge up front, just inhaling as much coffee as I possibly could to try to stay awake, when this old woman came walking in. She was holding this itty-bitty dog in one arm, and with her other hand she was carrying one of those blue tins that those sugar cookies come in around Christmas time.

Registration asked if the woman needed to be seen, to which the woman replied, "Me? Oh, I hope not."

Registration asked the woman if she needed to visit, to which the woman replied, "Well, no."

I couldn't help but to do an internal eye roll. I couldn't help it. I was exhausted, and everyone was getting on my last nerve. I actually considered faking an injury so they'd make me go home. I didn't care about overtime or any of that. Whenever I had to speak to my coworkers or management, part of me wanted to puff my chest out and say, "Fire me. I dare you."

Now, there's no real polite way to say, "If you don't need to be seen and you're not here to visit a patient, can you tell me what it is that you want from the emergency room?"

The registration person was new, though, and she didn't have a lot of tact, so that's pretty much how the question came out of her mouth. I choked on my coffee and thought I was going to die. I ended up spilling half of what was left in my cup all over my scrubs, so that was just another thing to add to my list of things that would absolutely go wrong on that day because the universe hates me.

The old woman placed her dog on the counter.

"Ma'am," I said, "you can't have animals on the counter."

"He's not hurting anything," she gently protested.

"Ma'am," I said, "I'm sorry, but animals aren't even allowed in the hospital unless they're service animals."

The woman got huffy and said, "Well, if you're going to be so rude to me, fine."

She shoved the blue tin at the registration clerk and said, "I found that by the lake.

Remind me never to come to this hospital if I need anything."

The old woman then stormed off, complaining the entire way about how no other place in town ever complained about her dog being on the counters or in the businesses. I wasn't too heartbroken about it.

Now, at the time, I had pretty much forgotten all about the patient we'd started calling 'Stubby.' (Just to make it clear, his girlfriend started calling him that first, and it became a little joke between staff and the family, so it's not a name we just made up to mock the patient.)

I told registration, "Open it up. Let's find out what she brought us."

Registration held the tin in her elbow and yanked at the lid with her other hand. The lid was pretty stuck on there, so she handed it to me. Well, whenever I got the lid off, whatever was in the tin went flying out and went down my shirt.

Since I was so tired, I moved slowly and more concerned with taking another drink of coffee before I reached in my shirt and started fishing out whatever it was that went down it.

When I finally pulled the object from between my bra and my shirt, the registration girl screamed. People in back thought there was a dangerous situation up front by the screams they heard, so they hit the lockdown button, which set off strobe lights and tripped a silent alarm to notify security.

"Look at that," I said calmly. "It's a finger."

We knew that it was highly unlikely that the finger did *not* belong to our fireworks patient from the previous night, but none of the staff from that shift were on that morning (lucky them), so they made me call the police department to report that an elderly woman brought us a human finger in a cookie container. I mean, that doesn't sound alarming or sinister at all to report at nine in the morning, right?

I explained to officers what had happened the night before, but they wanted to double check with the old woman, so they reviewed our security footage and tracked her down by her license plate information. I guess she told them that she'd gone out for her morning walk and was feeding the ducks when her dog wandered a few feet away and was found chewing on something he'd found in the grass. That something just happened to be my patient's finger. No word on where the second one ended up, but I'm just guessing that an animal found it and carried it off.

Oh, get this: the old woman asked the officer if she could file a discrimination complaint against me because I had told her to get her dog off the counter.

I ended up going home two hours early that day, and I remember thinking the entire shift, "I don't get paid enough for this shit."

-T.J.P.
Kentucky

The Maury Show, ER Edition

I admit that I've always been a bit of a lady's man. My coworker told me to be honest with you and let you know that everyone at work calls me a man-whore.

Whatever it is that you call me, I guess it's all the same. I love women, and I love sex. I'm not some pig who loves 'em and leaves 'em. I am honest with the women I meet, and I won't have intercourse with anyone unless we're both in agreement that we just want to have a little fun with no strings attached.

I guess I should say that's all past-tense because that's basically how I was from the ages of 18 to 26. I got married a few months ago, and I love my wife. I've never cheated on her, and I'm not remotely interested in any other woman. Meeting my wife has changed everything about my life for the better. The funny thing is, is that we met when I was trying to pick up other women, ended up hitting it off and going back to her place, and we *didn't* sleep together for at least a month. We did get married pretty soon after we met, but when it's right it's right.

Anyway, last week I was having a day from hell. I swear, I don't think I've ever had a worse day at work.

Patients were flooding in, and they were all in bad condition. We received two separate MVAs back to back, and there had been fatalities in both accidents. We lost three more victims from both crashes. Two of them were children.

We were also receiving overdoses, domestic violence victims, and someone had pushed a woman out of a moving vehicle out front. That woman was found to have multiple stab wounds, and nobody could really tell who'd pushed her out of the car or remember a make and model for the car. Unfortunately, that woman died of her injuries, and we didn't even know who she was.

That's what hit me the hardest about that day, I think. I couldn't imagine dying as a John Smith like my patient died as a Jane Doe.

Well, I was up front, waiting for the insurance claim person to give me information for a patient in back, when this woman peeked through the glass and said, "John? Is that you?"

I honestly didn't know who the hell this woman was, but she was pretty and seemed to know who I was, so I just kind of smiled and said hi back.

"It's so good to see you again," she said.

"You, too."

"I've really been wanting to get into contact with you," she said. "If I would've known you worked here, I would've come told you a long time ago."

"Uh, told me what?" I asked.

The insurance rep gave me my paperwork and I stood up to excuse myself back to my patient.

"That I'm pregnant," the woman said.

I looked over, saw this woman's HUGE pregnant belly, and the room started spinning. For sure, I thought she had been one of the women I'd slept with right before I met my wife. All I could think about was having to tell my wife that some woman came to my job and told me that I was going to be a dad. And by the looks of it, I had maybe another week before I was going to be expected to change diapers.

Well, I did what any man in that situation would do, and I passed out.

I wasn't out for very long. I fell against the insurance claim rep's file cabinet, but by the time I hit the ground I was conscious again.

Everyone wanted me to stay calm and seated, but I couldn't stay calm when my one-night stand was at my job telling me she was pregnant.

I asked the woman if she'd step aside and talk to me. I told her, "I always use a condom. Did it break?"

She looked at me, wildly confused, and then asked, "You don't have any idea who I am, do you?"

I thought it was some kind of trick question, so I kind of laughed and said, "Sure I do… Jenny."

She gave me a dead-serious look and said, "My name is Jane. I can't believe you'd forget. That night was special to me."

At this point, I started panicking again, but the pregnant woman started laughing.

"Relax," she said. "You changed my tire on the freeway, remember?"

I didn't remember.

"I got sick, and I told you my husband and I were trying for a baby, but our doctor said he didn't know if we could."

"Oh, yeah!" I exclaimed. "I gave you that specialist's name because you guys just moved here."

"Yeah," she laughed. She patted her belly and said, "Twins!"

I let out this huge sigh of relief as I congratulated her.

"Don't worry," she joked, "you're not my kids' daddy or anything."

When I went home that evening, I told my wife all about the encounter. I made sure to tell her up front, though, "Babe, I wasn't the father, but..." before I told the rest of the story.

She and I didn't find it as amusing as all my coworkers did.

-Name and location withheld at request

My partner woke up from his nap while
we were staging, looked at me with a tired
expression, and asked, "You know how much
it'd suck to be a medic at Jurassic Park?"

-J.O.
Oregon

The Bee's Knees

I debated telling this story, but I figured so many people know already that what's a few more?

I was sitting outside on my porch a couple of days ago, and I was leaning forward in my chair because my back hurt. I remember my mom always telling me to be 'lady-like' and always make sure my legs were closed and my ankles were crossed, but it felt so much more comfortable to have my legs wide open as I scrolled through my cell phone.

I felt something crawl into my vagina, and I started panicking. I couldn't very well insert my fingers into my vagina as I was sitting on the front porch, so I jumped out of my seat with every intention of going inside. That's when I felt a sharp pain just inside my vagina.

I won't lie. I cried. I also screamed.

I could still feel something moving inside of me, so I panicked and called 911. Two paramedics showed up and took me to the emergency room, where they had me labeled as a vaginal pain complainant. I guess the paramedics forgot to tell the emergency room staff that I was pretty sure I'd been stung by a bee or wasp, because I could hear everyone talking about wasting their time with such a stupid complaint.

The doctor came in and performed a vaginal exam. He confirmed what I already knew: a bee had flown up my shorts and had made its way into my vagina. I guess it freaked out when I stood up, so it stung me.

Luckily, the doctor was able to use a pair of tweezer-looking things and remove the large bee from my vagina. He did his best to remove the stinger from my vaginal cavity, and he told me there wasn't much else he could do. I've never been so embarrassed in my life.

I think the doctor was embarrassed, too, because after he extracted the bee, I said to him, "Sorry to waste your time with such a stupid complaint."

The doctor turned red and apologized in a mumbled whisper.

I did feel like the sting hurt worse in my vagina than it's ever felt on my foot or arm. The rest of the side effects from a bee sting were/are the same. I have extreme itchiness and discomfort, along with a huge bump that I can feel with my fingers.

I'm the only one I've ever known to be stung inside the vagina by a bee, and I have a $3,000 hospital bill from my emergency room visit and ambulance ride to prove it. Lucky me.

-K.C.
Louisiana

If Your Friends Jumped off a Bridge...

I wish your books were around before I retired, because my coworkers and I could have probably kept you going on our stories alone. This story happened decades ago, so I don't remember all the details, but I remember the basics. Let's just say we were all beside ourselves when EMS brought the patient in.

It was the hottest day of the year and nobody wanted to be out in the heat, but back in the day you didn't have much of a choice because you were either a hardworking adult, or your parents didn't want to put up with you, so they sent you outside and told you not to come home until the street lights came on.

In our town, we didn't have a city pool, but we did have a river. That river was always packed in summer. We'd inflate inner tubes and tie them together before floating a few miles down. There was always a crowd, but we all knew how to have fun. I remember one young man always lugged his guitar along, and he'd give us a mini concert. Every now and then there'd be a fight, but it was rare. We were all too hot to be messing with that nonsense.

Anyway, while my coworkers and I were on shift and were dying in this cooped-up ED, I suppose the river scene was booming.

Our sheriff was actually the one to notify us that something was happening. He called over the radio and said, "Better start calling around, Jane. This isn't looking good for anyone."

He kept telling me that it was 'so bad,' but he kept getting distracted, so we didn't know for sure what to expect.

Six to eight minutes later, we met the ambulance at the back entrance. This was back when we didn't have the ambulances we have now. This one, I remember quite well, was a Bonneville, and it was the town's pride and joy because it was almost brand new. Blood leaked out of the back of the ambulance when they opened the doors. They'd manage to get the patient's ankle to stop bleeding, by using a tourniquet and attempting to bandage it to hold pressure, but the patient was bleeding profusely from his face, ears, nose, and mouth.

There is no doubt in my mind, that had this patient's medic crew not been half made up from war veterans, that he would have died from his injuries before arriving to our ED.

My coworker had enlisted as a nurse several years back, but even she was disgusted, so that can probably give you an idea of what we were dealing with.

"What happened out there?" our doctor shouted. "We're not equipped to treat these wounds."

"You'd better get him to someone who is then," one of the medics said, "'cause he's barely hanging on."

"What happened?" someone asked.

"He jumped from the bridge," the medic replied.

At the time, I'd never seen anything like this, but later we learned the details. The patient had heard about returning soldiers performing daredevil jumps off the bridge by using paracord to tie off.

Thinking he could do the same, our patient used brown twine rope, with one end tied around his ankle and the other tied to the bridge.

When our patient jumped, the force almost removed his foot at the location where the rope was tied. He then swung back and smacked face-first against one of the bridge pillars. The rope then snapped, and the patient landed on some rocks under the bridge.

We were able to get the patient transferred to a hospital in the city, which was about 45-minutes away, and our doctor made my coworker ride with him. I packed her a bag with a suture kit and bandages, just to attempt to control the patient's bleeding during transport.

What the patient attempted is now known as 'bungee jumping,' and it's not something I would ever do after seeing my patient's injuries. He lost his foot at the ankle and sustained broken bones to his face, dislocated his hip, broke his back, and suffered from internally bleeding from his impact to the pillar.

Thankfully, the patient lived, but he was not in good spirits after the accident, and I don't think his life turned around for several years after that incident. He was left paralyzed from the accident.

-C.E.

Location withheld at request

<u>Oh, Man</u>

My sister went in labor, so she asked me to watch her twins after school. This meant I had to go pick the kids up from school, and it was my first time setting foot in there since I went to school there. I was pretty stoked to be in the building.

The boys were hanging out with their friends in their classroom, since they couldn't be released until I showed ID and signed some kind of paper.

When we were walking out, some jackass kid purposely but 'accidentally' ran into one of the boys and then taunted the boys by saying, "Bet you can't do this," before he leapt from the top of the staircase, soared over 11 steps, and landed flawlessly at the base of the staircase.

I could tell the boys were really feeling upset because of this creep, so I thought I'd be the cool uncle and jump off the stairs.

Guess what?

I didn't land as graciously as that bully did, and I had an idea that I wasn't going to as I was flying through the air with my arms flapping and my legs kicking.

What happened, you ask?

They had to call 911, that's what happened.

I ended up having to get seven staples to close the gash in my head, and I snapped my ankle. That required surgery, so I had to call my brother-in-law, and while he was in the ER, calling around to see if one of the family's neighbors could watch the boys, my niece decided that would be a perfect time to come shooting out, even though my sister had already been in labor for 13 hours.

Yeah, I'm the asshole who made my brother-in-law miss the birth of his third child.

I felt absolutely horrible because he was in the military when the twins were born, so he missed their births during a deployment.

They ended up having another kid two years later and I was still feeling so bad about making my brother-in-law miss my niece's birth that I gave them a $500 gift card to Babies 'R' Us.

-O.M.
Missouri

OMG

I've read all of your books and have seen where a lot of people have talked about having bad days at work. I'd like to share what my worst day at work looked like. Let me warn you that it's not gonna be pretty.

My husband and I both work in ERs at different hospitals. Because of this, we are huge fans of meal prep, so on our days off we take turns making dinner, packing them in individual containers, and stacking them in the fridge. Each night, we place our water bottles in the fridge, so we'll have cold water available. We each start out with one bottle of flavored water poured into our bottles, and then we both end up refilling our water bottles with tap water at least three times per shift.

I guess I forgot to set my alarm, so when I woke up I realized I would be late for work if I didn't leave right then. I had to skip my shower, had to go to work with no makeup on, and I had my hair up in a ratty ponytail. I was putting my scrub top on as I was going down the stairs, missed a step, and fell down the rest of them.

We'll count waking up late and falling down the stairs as reasons one and two of why my night sucked.

I didn't even have time to say goodbye to my husband, who was in the computer room playing video games. I was a little upset about this because by the time I got home, he would be gone to have his colonoscopy that next morning. I was scheduled to go in early the next day, too, so we wouldn't see each other for a day, practically.

I only had time to grab my water bottle and a Tupperware container from the fridge, grab my purse/keys, and head out the door.

On the way to work, my 'low fuel' light came on. I figured I'd just refuel in the morning, so I pulled in the parking lot, parked 12,000 miles away from the ER, and I slipped and fell on ice twice as I was trying to get inside.

The 'low fuel' light wasn't that bad, but it was annoying, so let's say that and slipping on ice became reasons three, four, and five of why my night was horrible.

Upon clocking in, I realized we were short-staffed. That's always fun. (Reason number six, if you're keeping track.)

I knew I wasn't going to have a lot of time to eat or drink, so I chugged my water and got to work. In hindsight, I guess the texture was a bit off, but we'd just bought new brands of flavored water, so I thought maybe that had something to do with it.

Busy, busy, busy.

MVAs, flu-like symptoms, runny noses, Alt LOCs, leg pains, hip pains, falls…You name it, we had it check in. It was pure chaos.

Just when I thought it couldn't get any worse, a drug seeker ran through our station and attacked my coworker. The two wrestled for a minute, before a tech and doctor could pull the patient off my coworker. My coworker works out often and actually does MMA-style fighting on weekends, so he was completely fine.

My dinner, on the other hand, was not fine. The container got knocked off the counter during the scuffle, and my chicken breast and grilled vegetables were smashed all over the floor.

I'm going to go ahead and say that the patient flow to RN ratio and my dinner being ruined can count as reasons seven and eight of why my night was the worst.

We received an unexpected code as a walk in. Technically, this woman's boyfriend carried her inside. She wasn't breathing, and she had no pulse. Her boyfriend said she shot up in the car on the way home from their dealer's house. What's worse about all that is that the woman's child was in the car and was old enough to realize that mommy took drugs and wasn't breathing.

I was in the room, pounding away at chest compressions, when my stomach gurgled.

"Not now," I whispered, hoping I could tell my body to hold off.

My stomach gurgled again, and before I could even make sense of what was going on, I had explosive diarrhea. It ran out of my underpants, soaked my scrub bottoms, ran down my legs, and was all over the floor.

If you think that's bad, let me tell you that I couldn't stop doing compressions, and my diarrhea didn't stop, either.

Someone finally pushed me out of the way and told me to go take care of myself, and I had to powerwalk out of the room and towards the nearest bathroom while *everyone* I encountered stared and talked about me.

I reached the employee bathroom just as my stomach gurgled again, but I couldn't get in.

"Just a second," someone said from inside.

I banged on the door so hard that I felt the crunch in my finger before I felt the pain. "I don't have a minute!" I screamed.

I couldn't help it. I relieved myself *again* in my pants. On top of that, I could tell my finger was broken.

At this point, I was sobbing, and I didn't know what to do. I turned around and was trying to remember where the next nearest bathroom was. There was a trail of diarrhea leading to me, and I was so embarrassed that I wished I could turn invisible. I had no idea why I was so sick all the sudden, especially when all I had to drink was flavored water. (We're going to count the code and diarrhea as reasons nine, 10, 11, and 12.)

A coworker ran up to me and helped me get to the decon shower. I couldn't stop the diarrhea, and I felt disgusting. It was so bad and startled my coworker so much that she paged any available physician to come down to the ER to talk to me about anything I had ingested or possible illnesses I had come in contact with.

"Hello?!" I screamed at one of the physicians from ICU, "I work in the emergency room. I come in contact with illnesses every day!"

That doctor told me to sign in as a patient, so I did and had to sit on a potty chair while I waited for someone to come see me. I knew it was going to take a while because they were still working on that code and had received an SNF 912.

I managed to get in my purse while I was waiting, and when I turned on my phone, I had six missed calls and several text messages from my husband.

"Did U take the bottle w/ the purple lid?" one of the messages read.

I scrolled down.

"Don't drink it!"

"U took my golytely."

"Calling u now."

"Answer ur phone."

"Pick up."

"DON'T DRINK THE WATER!"

I was so mad and embarrassed that I screamed out, "Are you fucking kidding me?!" at the top of my lungs and I threw my phone across the room.

That was a particularly bad move because my phone broke.

I was going to call my husband to take me home.

My husband had just gotten a new phone number the day before, and the only place I had it 'written down' was in the phone I had just smashed to pieces. (Reasons 13, 14, and 15.)

I was hooked up to an IV and basically was told that I was 'lucky' that I hadn't drank 'that much' of it, after I showed the doctor my water bottle. I kept getting sick, and they said I must have a hypersensitivity to it.

I had to call my sister to come pick me up, and I had to wear an adult diaper home because I was still experiencing diarrhea.

When I got home, my husband was on the toilet, which was the ONLY toilet we had, so I had to use the trash can.

It turns out, my husband TRIPLED the dosage of his GoLytely and mixed it with flavored water. He mixed the rest in another bottle once he realized he had either misplaced the other bottle or I had taken it. I could have killed that man that night.

I felt a lot better after another two or three hours, but only physically. I called my supervisor that night and told her I needed to request the next day off. I said, "because," and was going to explain, but she cut me off and said she already knew what happened, and that I could take off as much time as I needed. I felt so bad about what happened at work that I felt obligated to buy housekeeping flowers and I didn't make eye contact with my coworkers for about two shifts after I returned to work.

That mix-up cost me my dignity and professional reputation for a long while. On top of that, the phone I ruined was under contract and the warranty didn't cover that kind of damage, so I had to pay $800 for a new phone.

My husband ended up being fine, by the way, but he complained and whined about his colonoscopy for a week. Buddy, I don't even feel bad for you, after the night I had.

-Name and location withheld at request

That's Your Own Fault, Dude

I was at this party one night, when I saw this gorgeous woman standing across the room. I didn't think I had a shot with her, but I figured the worst thing that could happen is I'd ask her out and she'd tell me to get lost.

Well, imagine my surprise when we just hit it off and she said she would LOVE to go out with me the next night! I was ecstatic.

This woman was so beautiful that when she suggested we go ice skating for our first date, I was too scared to tell her that I really didn't know *how* to ice skate. I decided I'd wait until the date and tell her that I hadn't skated in years, and maybe she'd take pity on me and cut me a break.

Yeah, so the next day came and I picked her up. She brought her own skates and when she asked where mine were, I lied and said someone had broken into my car and took the box that I'd thrown them in. She seemed to buy that.

We got to the rink and I rented a pair of skates. She was already out on the ice as I was lacing up, and it was obvious she'd been skating from a young age or had at least spent a lot of her adult life skating because she was a pro at it. She was twirling and doing crap you see on the Olympics.

I made up every excuse that I could not to go out on that ice, but she was getting pretty insistent, so I eased out.

At first, it wasn't that bad. I slipped a little bit, but I played it off as I was wearing cheap rental skates.

She started doing circles around me and wanted me to skate with her, so of course I wasn't going to tell her no.

I should have told her no because when I tried to pick up speed, I ended up falling, doing the splits, and on the way down I caught my head on the railing around the rink. The manager at the rink called 911 and the rest of our first date was spent with this woman being kind enough to text my mother for me.

I ended up getting seven staples to my head, and they said I had a concussion. Luckily, I didn't injure my penis or testicles.

Get this: my date told me it was painfully obvious that I was lying about being able to skate, but she just wanted to see how far I'd go to keep the lie going before I came clean!

Moral of the story? Tell the truth from the beginning, and then maybe you won't end up in the ER on your first date.

We've been dating for a year now, and she doesn't know it, but we're going back to that rink tonight, where I'm proposing to her.

-K.L.
New York

Riding the Waves

I think it was about 03:00 when a male patient waddled to my triage desk and told me he needed to be seen. When I asked for his chief complaint, he told me he only wanted to speak to a male.

"Sir," I said, "I need to enter a complaint here, or I can't continue to register you."

"My butt hurts," he mumbled.

I had to go down the line of standard triage questions. After establishing the patient's drug, alcohol, and medical history, I began asking him questions about his chief complaint.

"Would you say the pain is throbbing, achy, or a sharp pain?"

"Uhhhhh," he said.

"Does it hurt if you move a particular way, or is it constant?"

"Um," he thought. "Uh, it's constant."

"And do you remember when the pain started?" I asked.

He said, "Well, my girlfriend left around midnight, and I watched some TV, so maybe around two?"

"Have you recently fallen or sustained trauma to that region?"

He turned bright red.

"Sir," I assured him, "you can't tell me anything I haven't heard before."

He hesitated before whispering, "I may or may not have something stuck up there."

"What did you stick up there?" I asked.

"A knick-knack," he told me.

"A knick-knack?"

He nodded. "You know, like a little guy."

He started waving his hands. "It's a guy, but I'm not gay. I swear, I'm not gay."

I blinked and then said, "Sir, nobody's accusing you of anything. Even if you were gay, none of us would care, especially not me. Both of my sons are gay, and I still love them."

"Well," he snapped, "I'm not a homo."

I clearly rolled my eyes within the patient's view, and then I guided him to an examination room.

We didn't have any male nurses on staff that night, so I had to skip straight to the doctor and fill him in. The doctor sighed and entered the room. A few minutes later, we heard screaming. Then, the doctor called out for any available nurse.

I entered the room and was in charge of holding the patient's hand while the doctor tried again to remove the knick-knack from the patient's rectum.

The patient screamed bloody murder.

After a few more minutes, the doctor ordered the patient be sent to X-ray, so we could see the shape and position of the knick-knack. The film showed a 7"H, 5"W figurine lodged almost sideways in the patient's rectum. Because of its size and positioning, the doctor concluded he could not remove it, so he asked me to schedule the patient for surgery.

When I explained to the patient that he would be sent to surgery, he cried. When I asked if he wanted me to call his girlfriend, he shouted and cursed at me. I left the room.

Surgery called down a little later and said they retrieved a figurine of a pirate surfing on a wave, holding a treasure chest in one hand and some type of weapon in the other. The wave was actually part of the figurine.

Aside from being confused as to why the patient would stick this up his butt, I couldn't help but to wonder who would want that kind of figurine on display in his or her home.

-B.R.

Georgia

You're on Your Own

As much as I love being a nurse, I sometimes hate it just as much. I suppose I don't hate being a nurse as much as I hate some of the unwanted attention it brings. My family always seems to find *some* way to announce that I'm a nurse, even when nobody cared or asked. My friends always hit me up for advice. It can get crazy.

My friend wanted me to go to this guy's apartment with her. She seemed to mistake my being single with being lonely, which I absolutely was not because I was secretly dating someone. I just didn't want everyone to know about it at the time.

Anyway, I agreed to go to the apartment with my friend because I knew they'd all start drinking, and I didn't want to leave my friend drunk and alone with strangers.

When we got to the apartment, there were a bunch of guys there. Most of them were drunk and playing video games. The music was loud, and I could smell pot.

Everyone kept hitting on me and trying to get me to drink, so I just sat in a chair in the corner and played on my phone while my friend was doing shots.

I guess about an hour had passed and my friend started whining that she was hungry, so the guy trying to get in her pants said he'd go make her some pizza rolls.

Well, I saw the light burn out as soon as he flipped the switch, so I figured he'd continue to make pizza rolls with the light off. I mean, it wasn't exactly rocket science to turn on the oven and stick a baking sheet in there, right? And there was more than enough light coming from the other rooms for him to see what he was doing. I'm guessing he didn't think of any of this because he was also highly intoxicated.

"Guys," he announced to the friends who weren't listening to him, "I need a chair."

"Your mom's a chair," someone yelled to him.

"That doesn't even make sense," I muttered.

"Jane," I begged, "can we go?"

"No! John's gonna make me food. Here, you should get to know Jason."

"I don't want to get to know Jason," I said with a sigh. "I'm tired and want to leave."

"After my food," my friend said.

I sighed again.

For a few minutes, John wandered around the apartment, presumably looking for a chair or ladder. Unfortunately, he couldn't find one, so the next thing I knew, this 200-something-pound man was dragging a cat tower across the apartment.

Sensing an accident that I certainly didn't want to tend to, I warned, "Don't do that."

"I'm fine," he replied.

"You may be fine now, but that's not gonna hold you. You're gonna get hurt."

Jane giggled and said, "But you're a nurse, silly."

"I'm A nurse," I said. "I'm not HIS nurse."

"I won't get hurt," John said.

I'm sure you can guess that John did get hurt. In fact, as soon as John climbed on the cat tower, the whole thing collapsed, and he landed on top of the stove. His head bounced off this half-wall that divided the kitchen area from a dining area, and he was not only bleeding, but he was also unconscious.

Everyone freaked out and told me to do something, so I called 911 and then checked John for a pulse. I was careful not to move him too much, and I instructed the only other sober person there to wait downstairs for EMS. I did my best to stop the bleeding, but it was clear John required medical attention.

I didn't want to go to the ER, but Jane was panicking, so we went to the waiting room, where my mom just happened to be because her friend was experiencing coronary symptoms.

My mom saw us in the waiting room and ran up to us, almost crying, because she thought we were hurt or sick.

Jane gets extra chatty when she's drunk, so she told my mom about how she was trying to hook me up with Jason.

Of course, my mom got all excited because she's been trying to get me to date for years, right?

I couldn't get the two to calm down, so I finally just screamed out, "Mom! I'm a lesbian, okay?"

Jane laughed and punched my shoulder. She said, "You are not."

I had to come clean in the waiting room—the busy waiting room, where everyone around us watched like they were at a live taping of Jerry Springer—that I had been secretly dating a tech from Oncology for at least six months and that our relationship was so serious that when I was talking about moving in with her, it wasn't just a roommate situation like my mom and Jane thought it was.

My mom started freaking out because she was raised in a religious household and thinks being gay is okay unless you're her family members. Otherwise, being gay is definitely not an option.

Well, my mom started having a meltdown so bad that security came and told us we'd have to leave if she couldn't tone it down. She couldn't help herself, though, so I had to sign her in for a panic attack, and she ended up with an oxygen cannula and an Ativan drip.

My mom ended up being fine and she got over my bombshell. Jane dated John for two or three months, but then he got drunk at her family's Thanksgiving and puked on her mom's Pomeranian, so that relationship didn't last long.

-A.R.

Virginia

<u>Hey, Fellas</u>

Earlier that day, a hot girl wrote her number on a piece of paper, and I shoved that paper in my pocket.

I was walking through the park a little later, when I reached in my pocket for my cigarettes. When I pulled out my cigarettes, the piece of paper got caught in the wind and blew to the other side of this tall fence thing. The pillars were concrete, and the fence part was wrought iron. There was a gravestone and a monument on the other side, so I guess they put the fence thing around it to keep people out.

Anyway, I couldn't climb over this thing, so I thought maybe I could reach through it enough to grab the piece of paper. It blew away, so I kept forcing myself through the metal spools.

I still couldn't reach the piece of paper, and I realized I was stuck. No matter how much I squirmed, I just couldn't free myself.

Thankfully, an elderly man called the fire department. They had to come and cut the spools because they couldn't get me out, either.

I was so worried about the piece of paper with that girl's phone number on it that I lunged forward instead of backwards when the fire department cut me loose.

The paper that blew away wasn't even the one the girl wrote on. *That* piece of paper was in my *other* pocket. I felt so dumb.

I think it was about a month later that I received a bill in the mail. It was from the city, charging me for damaging city property. They made me pay $611 as a fine and to help repair the fence thing.

The worst part of all of this is that I did call the number that girl had given me.

It was to a local pizza place.

-S.O.
New Jersey

Tough Love

When the nurse asked me how I got my bloody nose and busted lip, I thought I'd rather lie to her and say I got beaten in a fight, than explain I stepped on a garden hoe to test my reflexes on the stick.

My reflexes are apparently not that great because I had to get two stitches to close my lip, and they said I was lucky I didn't break my nose with how much blood was coming out of it.

The bad part is that my grandma was watching me from the kitchen window and right before I hurt myself, she yelled, "I'm not taking you to the hospital if you hurt yourself."

And she didn't. She sent grandpa out to tell me I was stupid and hand me my car keys.

-P.Y.
Nevada

Studying is Dangerous

I was at the station during a 24-hour stretch, and I was trying to study for my upcoming nursing exams. Throughout the night, I hadn't been able to get much done in terms of studying because every time I'd sit on the couch and pull out my books, someone would call 911 for a stubbed toe or something equally frivolous.

When we got back from our latest call, I announced that I was going to the bunker room, where we have a bunch of bunk beds to catch up on rest.

I thought I could be slick and slip my textbook under the slats of the bunk above me, and then my hands would be free to take notes. I was a genius!

The second the book slipped, I realized I was not a genius. My book weighed six pounds. It landed on my face. I got up to inspect myself in a mirror and noticed my eye was already swollen and my skin was blackening from the bruising. Yeah, I gave myself a black eye.

I was so angry because I was supposed to take engagement pictures with my fiancée the next day, that my anger got the best of me and I kicked this raggedy box that was next to the door.

I immediately regretted that decision.

The long story short is that I gave myself a black eye and then broke my foot in two places when I kicked that box.

I was put on light duty at work for a few months, and I had to cross the stage on crutches when I finally passed my nursing exam.

Talk about embarrassing.

-O.P.
Pennsylvania

Extreme Measures

The front porch of my rental house has nails coming loose from the boards, and then the concrete stairs are uneven. Since I've lived here, all my friends and visitors know that I am extra paranoid about someone getting hurt by tripping on the nails or falling down the stairs, so I warn people 800 times when they come over.

Guess what?

Last winter I tripped over one of the nails, fell down the stairs, and broke my arm.

My friends thought it was hilariously ironic that I spent so much time warning others that my porch was dangerous, yet I was the one who fell and got hurt.

I sent my hospital bill to my landlord because he'd been telling me for over a year that he was going to fix the issues. He paid, and I got a new porch and steps.

I guess that was one way to really get his attention, so now whenever I tell him there's a problem with the house, he rushes right over to fix it.

-N.G.

New Hampshire

A Man of Constant Sorrow

My husband invited a bunch of friends over to drink and watch football, and they all got there right as I was leaving for work. I work at the ED in our local hospital, and my shifts for the rest of the week were overtime, so I was exhausted before I even made it out the door.

I kissed my husband goodbye and jokingly told him I didn't want to see him in my ED.

About two hours after I clocked in, who do you think showed up as a patient? If you guess my husband, you win a cookie.

When our living room light bulb burned out, my drunk and idiot of a husband climbed up on a chair and attempted to change the light bulb.

What my husband did not do was turn the ceiling fan off first, so he got clocked in the forehead and the back of his head, before he fell off the chair and nearly severed his ear from his head.

After more than 20 sutures and after being told to remain in a lying position, but husband sat up and whacked his head on the overhead light the doctor had used to better see my husband's wound. The light bar gashed part of the sutures open and left a deep cut on the other side of my husband's forehead. The doctor had to come back in and sew my husband up for a second time.

My husband was discharged from the ED and went to jump down from the table (even after he was told not to), and he collapsed as soon as he hit the ground, screaming of pain.

He had somehow broken his foot.

At this point, I just told Charge I needed to go home to make sure my husband didn't decapitate himself trying to get inside.

I think they were so tired of him by the time we got him discharged (again) three hours later, that Charge was okay with me leaving, but only because that meant I'd take my husband with me.

When I got home, I saw the house was a disaster. So, not only did I have to put up with my husband acting like he'd been run over by a bus, but I also had to clean up the entire mess that he and his friends made.

-L.R.
Ohio

It Keeps Getting Worse

I work in at a pediatrician's office as a secretary. I never worry about job security because people are always having kids, and there will never be a shortage of worrisome mothers flipping the hell out because their kid somehow got a jelly bean stuck in his or her ear.

I had a particularly difficult family member who'd come in to get a child treated for a rash. This woman stated she was a family friend, but she couldn't provide any documentation that she had permission to have any sort of custody of the child, nor could she provide the child's date of birth. I stated that until she could come back with the proper paperwork, we could not sign the child into our office.

The woman asked for a piece of paper and a pen. She stated she was going to run outside and call the child's mother. When I told her that I would also need to speak with the mother, she said she would come inside once they finished their discussion.

In a hurry to get the woman out of my way so I could answer the phone, I yanked my supply drawer open and started doing a very audible hissing sound because I somehow whacked myself in the ribs with the drawer.

I then removed a pen and tried to hand it to the woman, but I dropped it and the pen rolled under my desk.

I'm the queen of being lazy. In fact, if I had been at home when I did that, I would have used my monkey toes to hand the pen to myself. Instead, I figured I could lean forward and grab the pen from the floor, without ever having to leave my office chair.

Well, I tried to reach the pen, but I just needed to lean a *little* more forward. When I did that, I fell out of my chair and hit my mouth on the wooden footrest my husband had purchased for me. I felt a sharp, stabbing pain that quickly became a throbbing pain, and I felt something loose in my mouth. I spit the object into my palm and realized I had broken one of my front teeth.

I tried to jump up, but in a panic, I forgot I had left my supply drawer open. I whacked the top of my head against t he drawer so hard that my vision blurred, and I felt dizzy.

"Are you okay?" the woman at the desk asked.

"I'm okay," I said with a nervous chuckle. I put my hand upon the top of my head and said, "Probably gonna bruise, that's all."

I then felt something on my hand, so I looked, and my palm and fingers were covered in blood. The woman at the desk saw this, too, so she fainted. Everyone in the waiting room panicked and started screaming, so imagine having a horrible day and then adults and a bunch of toddlers start shrieking in fear. Yeah, not really a great time.

Someone called 911 and two ambulances transported the woman and me to the emergency room.

Thankfully, the woman was fine. She never wanted to go to the emergency room anyway, but my boss pretty much insisted that she went, so she was nice enough to listen.

I, on the other hand, received eight staples, had a concussion, and I had to schedule an emergency appointment with my dentist, who decided the best thing to do would be to fit me with a crown.

Spoiler alert: It wasn't the kind of crown I wanted.

-J.D.

Indiana

Q & A

I have received many messages from readers, and I figured answering questions I often receive could replace the traditional 'Message to Readers' I've used to end my previous books. Here we go.

Q: Have you received submissions about [high-profile news]? Where are those stories?

A: Yes, I have. I privately respond to all messages, but I will not ask to use anyone's stories that pertain to mass shootings, terrorism, political activism, or any news that is so high-profile. I choose this for several reasons.

First of all, that stuff isn't entertainment. It's tragedy. I understand some of the stories you've read in my books are heartbreaking, but if I do use sad stories in my books, I usually try to choose the stories that contain lessons or will encourage a reader to be smarter, kinder, or more thoughtful of themselves and/or others.

Secondly, high-profile news stories are almost impossible to edit so that people can't find specifics of the incident online or from news sources. I realize that kind of sounds like, 'So you *would* use those stories if you *could,*' but that is not the case whatsoever. I would not use those stories because I'm disgusted by what I see in the news, and I'm sure you are, too. But, even if I could use the stories, I would never jeopardize anyone's identity through these submissions or any of my own stories, and especially in high-profile cases, it's unlikely that someone won't be able to be identified later on.

Writing about someone's local happenings is a little different than reporting on something that made international news. If I ever discuss high-profile events, I'll have to take a lot of time to ask myself if the lesson in the story outweighs the impact it has made on millions of people around the globe.

■■■■■■■■■■■■■■■■■■■■■■■■■■■■■■■■■■■■■

Q: What do you while we're waiting for another book?

A: Pretend I'm working. No, seriously, I do try to work a little each day. I often work on (non-medical) books I'm not sure I'll ever finish. I do some freelance transcription on the side (very rarely medical topics... I mostly transcribe interviews and legal matters.), and then whenever I'm sick of working or just don't want to work in general, I play video games, run errands, or do stuff around the house (clean, read, lounge around).

I do not have traditional working hours, but I still work. Right now, it's 04:18, and I'm trying to get this book finished so you guys can have it sooner than I had planned. I probably won't go to bed until 05:00 or later, and I'll probably wake up around 10. From there, I take care of my pets and get right back to work.

■■

I take days off from all work every now and then, but I'm usually doing *some* kind of work to stay busy and pay bills.

■■■

Q: I follow you on social media. Why don't you ever talk about [MeToo, politics, racial divide]? Don't you care?

A: There's a time and place for everything, and for me, that's usually not on my public social media. I very highly doubt you want to go to the drive-thru at Wendy's and hear your cashier rant about sexual harassment, Congress, and constitutional rights. I will occasionally mention something and touch down on my feelings about the subject matter, but in case you guys haven't noticed, the internet isn't really tolerant and inviting of opinions.

Yes, I *do* care about what's going on in the world. Yes, I am angry about what I see. Yes, some news stories make me cry.

I care, I really do. But I also care about creating a welcoming environment to all of my readers, regardless of their own opinions of these topics. I feel that while we're discussing how stupid some of the people in the world can be, for a brief minute we're all at peace from everything going on around us.

Q: Have you ever considered becoming a nurse or joining the EMS field?

A: A thousand times over, no. And you guys wouldn't want me as your nurse or medic, either. For starters, I suck at math, so I'd probably never be able to even pass the math course for medication doses.

Secondly, have any of you been paying attention to these books? HA! I use humor to mask every negative emotion I experience. If you come to me in tears, I might be able to hold it together for a few minutes, but eventually, I'm going to make a twisted joke and end up a hashtag.

When I worked around patients and family members in need, I often came home and coped with my emotions via unhealthy vices.

I'm not a very social person when the option to stay home alone is concerned, so I need time to recharge after any type of social encounter. It's just not in my blood to enter any long-term career where I have to be in direct contact with a large number of people on a constant basis, especially when emergent situations pile on emotions pertaining to death or illness.

Also, I can't handle puke, as most of you are aware. That reason alone is enough of a reason to never consider a caretaker position.
▪▪

Q: Do you miss working at the hospital?

A: I miss most of my former coworkers and being able to assist those in need. I also miss carry-ins and when the guy from the gas station came over at closing and brought us all the potato wedges he couldn't sell.
▪▪

Q: Why are your books so expensive? Do you really think $2.99 is a fair price?

A: The same people complaining about the price of my books probably don't bat an eye at spending $6 on a coffee.

Trust me, nobody understands 'the struggle' more than I do, which is exactly why the Kindle versions of my books are priced between 99-cents and $3.99. I don't recall ever pricing Kindle versions higher than $3.99.

For paperbacks, I am bound by a minimum listing price set by the publisher. This cost covers printing, distribution, and whatever other costs the publisher and listing websites charge on that side of things. I usually bump up the price from the minimum by a few cents to about a dollar, depending on the royalty calculator provided by the publisher. It's just enough to keep me out of the red. On paperbacks, depending on where you purchase your copy, I rarely make more than a few cents for each copy sold.

I want to keep my books affordable because I understand how costly it can be to find something recreational. Additionally, compared to other books, my releases are often priced far under what other authors sell at. I know I couldn't afford to pay $10.94 for a Kindle book each time a new one came out, nor would I want to pay that much for an electronic copy.

I also have to consider my own needs when pricing. I'm not a millionaire or anything, and I'm not out to bleed anyone dry, I promise! I do need to eat, though, and it's kinda cool to have stuff like electricity and running water.

Long story short, yeah, I think my prices are fair, and I don't think my books are too expensive.

Q: Hey, can I get that person's contact information? I'd like to help them out or talk to them about their experiences.

A: No, no, no. Privacy is a HUGE deal for me, so I just can't do that. I have passed messages along once or twice, but I can't reveal identities or specific locations. If someone wants to tell his or her story as a standalone and then be in contact with people, that's great. I won't be involved in that, though. There's way too much risk associated with that kind of stuff, at least in my opinion.

Those are all the questions I could think of this time around. As usual, if you have any comments or questions, feel free to drop me a line on my Facebook page, and I'll try to get back to you as soon as possible.

Again, THANK YOU for reading and recommending me to your friends. I can't thank you all enough for your support!

Have a great day and stay safe!

Check me out on Twitter!

https://twitter.com/AuthorKerryHamm

You can also find me on Facebook, by searching for 'Author Kerry Hamm.'